PRAISE FOR LB CAMERON, MD

At the time of publication, no praise was forthcoming for the author or this book.

From Blood To Gas

A Novel for Doctors

L.B. Cameron, MD

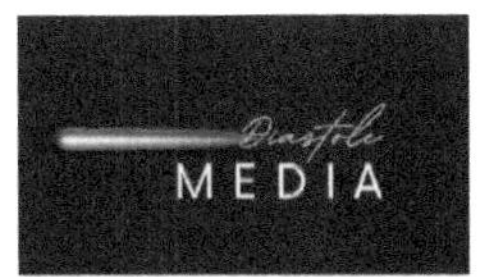

Copyright © 2025 by L.B. Cameron

All rights reserved.

No part of this publication may be reproduced, distributed, or transmitted in any form or by any means, including photocopying, recording, or other electronic or mechanical methods, without the prior written permission of the publisher, except as permitted by U.S. copyright law.

Cover and Interior Design by Diastole Media, LLC

Cover photo by Pascal Meier on Unsplash

ISBN 979-8-218-59823-5

Printed in the United States of America

First Edition

This book is a work of fiction. The story, all names, characters, and incidents portrayed in this production are fictitious. No identification with actual persons (living or deceased), places, buildings, and products is intended or should be inferred.

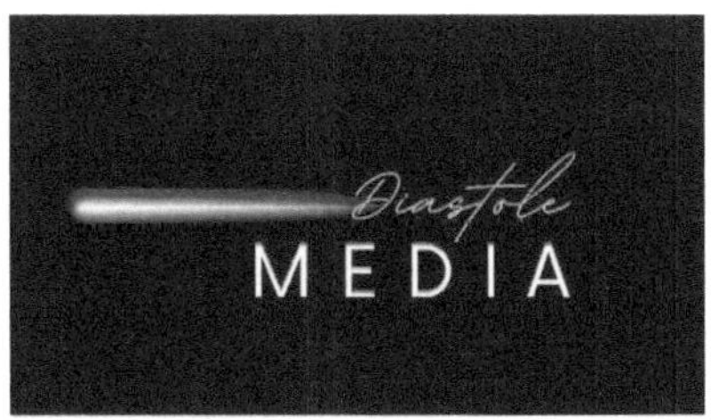

Dedication

This book is for all the imposters.
You know who you are.

PROLOGUE

You will never have a patient quite like your first.

The first patient will be different from the ones who come later, the ones who may harbor a hidden agenda or a secret contempt for you or an unspoken belief they are immortal. The first patient won't ask you too-personal questions or comment on your weight gain and ask when the baby is due. They won't shake your hand just a little too long, or call you diminutive nicknames, or stand blocking the door, or tell you how much they hate doctors with that look on their face like *don't you agree.* The first patient won't complain your appointments are too short, insisting upon an extra ten point five minutes that will cause every subsequent patient to complain you are running late. They won't wait until your hand is on the door to tell you the real reason they've come, the odd and visceral pain that's been eating at them for months. They won't bring you homemade jam every fall and learn your children's names and make your life so rich and so full, only to die of a cancer you missed on their last physical. They won't insist *it isn't your fault*, holding *your* hand to somehow comfort *you*, even though they are the one who is dying, only further proving the maxim that Nice People Die and Mean

People Live Forever, a real fact of medicine that will haunt you again and again and again and again. The other patients will do these things because they are (inconveniently, infuriatingly) flawed and human works in progress.

Not your first patient.

Your first patient will be simple, easy, complete. Your first patient will ask nothing of you. Your first patient will be *perfect*.

They can be this way because they are exquisitely and immutably and pre-existingly Already Dead. Expired. Passed away. Croaked. On to the great blue yonder. Kicked the bucket. A corpse or, as rebranded by the spin cycle of medical terminology, a *cadaver*. Previously Human, now Specimen, arriving dead and remaining dead for the duration of your relationship, assuming no vivifying lightning bolts or reanimating zombie viruses strike the lab during your tenure. They will lie in wait on your first day, perfectly still, the only one who will unwaveringly fulfill the titular implication of the word *patient*.

This first patient greets future doctors into the profession with shock and awe, as if facing the squish and the smell of death were a necessary precursor to someday preserving life. This initiation sets them into a lineage of medical grotesquerie that dates back to the days when apprentice physicians were tasked with robbing graves under the cover of night, before the advent of modern preservation techniques, when a strong stomach was necessary for the job. Now, today's pampered medical students get their bodies through more official channels, formalin-filled and refrigerated and inert, a far cry from the mad dash against decomposition the students of yore had to contend with. If one believes in ghosts, one must assume that every Gross Anatomy Lab is haunted by a physician from the 1700s, moaning into the darkness, *todaaaay's stuuuudents haaaave it toooooo eeeeeeasy.*

The modern day cadaver need not be snatched, thanks to body donors who gift themselves pre-mortem. These biological benefactors are often upper-middle-class, college-educated, erudite; the type of folks who have *an estate* they leave to the Nature Conservancy or a big name alma mater. They may write flowery notes as they lay in hospice waiting to die, notes sent along with their body to greet the students on day one. *Enjoy this gift and please make me proud. I know you'll make a great doctor someday.* They might make morbid little jokes like *let my wife know if you find a heart in there, she's not too sure,* or *give my face a little lift, will you?* They may apologize for the excessive adipose tissue overlying the gluteal muscles, *I know my husband didn't mind it but I hope it doesn't get in your way!* Jokes a dead person can make, because who is going to stop them. These bodies will have serene smiles frozen onto their still faces, like a macabre Mona Lisa, having died with the knowledge that their last earthly act will be this singular contribution to education.

Of course, not *every* first patient comes so willingly. Some arrive by way of estranged family members who were suddenly forced to contend with the final disposition of someone they either hated or hardly knew, and who discover body donation is a clever way to avoid the costs of cremation, and who otherwise have no particular horse in this race, except to say that *maybe this way Jack can actually contribute something to this world.* These reluctant bodies come without the serene smiles and sweet greetings, but they come with different surprises. The first patient can hold no secrets, not really, not so long as you hold a scalpel. Surprises, though? You can bet on it.

No matter the provenance, though, or what their animated existence was like, the first patient comes with one critical benefit — they can take no offense. You can curse at them softly under your breath while you work, bemoaning the redundant folds of scrotal tissue obscuring the cremaster. You can make crass jokes to your table partners about the size of their *corpus spongiosum* as your preceptors walk out of earshot. You can insult the sorry state of their stenotic and tortuous vasculature as they lay prone and beyond help; they won't complain. In that way, a dead person is a friend like no other. We should all be so lucky as to have one in our life for a time.

It's hard to appreciate this benefit in the moment. New medical students are too excited and nervous and preoccupied and busy and young and all the things that keep you from appreciating things in the moment. Years later, a doctor might think about this patient, wishing they had spent more time appreciating the artistry of the greater trochanter, or the brachial plexus, or the intersigmoid recess, wishing for a simpler time when the tasks were so palpable and defined. Wishing for a time when the end point had been predetermined, wishing the rest of medicine had such a precise and unchanging method laid out, a method that could be entombed in worn copies of lab manuals passing unchanged from student to student for 50 years without revision. While everything else changes on the same logarithmic scale as all facts in the Information Age, the dissection of a human body can remain static, having come to a point of perfection. There is a way. It is the way. The way does not change.

Sure, there is more than one way to skin a cat, the saying goes. (As if cat-skinning were a pastime popular enough to have a significant controversy between methods; a faction dedicated to hanging the creatures by their tails to skin ass-first, a head-first counterculture, a small and snobbish molecular gastronomy cohort who exchange various enzymatic self-skinning and preserving methods on the *r/catskinners* subreddit, you get the point). So, of course, there is more than one way to skin a cadaver as well. Every profession has its rebels and factions. The art of dissection has been around since at least the times of ancient Egypt, has lived through various periods of prohibition and exhibition, has come into the hands of such all-time greats as Galen and Vesalius. No doubt their way was quite different from ours, but the game was not the same in the earlier ages. They were catching as catch could back then, often charged with diving into, say, a partially decomposed leper in the unforgiving hot sun of the Roman summer.

Things are different now. Body dissection can now be undertaken at a slow and methodical pace, following a well-worn path of best practices honed by generations of students. Until the human form evolves beyond its current iteration, one need not second guess it. Each year, at each medical school, the first year students will undertake a task that echoes the efforts of last year's students, and the ones before them, and before them, and before them. The cadavers will wait for them in a standard repose, one that is documented in the manual, an unchanging tome written long ago by some man who has probably been, himself, long dead.

How will they find this preserved and perfect person? The hands will be wrapped in thin cloth, with the wrists tied together to prevent the arms from flopping off the edge of the table. The head will be shrouded, tied with loose twine around the neck, giving the body the appearance of someone who was taken hostage in the back of a van before landing in this cooled and well-lit laboratory for a long nap.

In death, the head and the hands are the parts too personal to reveal upfront. You have to earn those intimacies. You have to get to know your cadaver's sinew and heft, get desensitized to the act of flaying open their skin and running your fingers clumsily along the pathways of their vessels and nerves, desensitized to the formalin-fueled nightmares that come with such an intimate relationship with a dead person. You have to give them a name, tell stories with your lab partners about the life they lived and how they got those scars and whether they had ever been in love. Only then can you hold the hands that (hopefully) a loved one had held in the last moment of their life. Only then can you gaze upon the maybe-serene, maybe-surprised look on their stiffened face, frozen forever in its last conscious moment.

In life, we give our faces and our hands so willingly to the world. In death, it's better to start with the backside.

That's why the first act of patient care as a medical student, more often than not, will be to take the shrouded body, pull back the sheet (grimacing internally with the anticipation that the whole thing might sit bolt upright), and then roll them right over until they're tits-down. The backside provides a forgiving surface for the scalpel errors of an unskilled new student's hand, the big strap muscles easily palpable under the skin, thick and coarse from a lifetime of providing protection from unexpected blows that might come from behind. You can't start at the intimate top, nor the delicate extremities, nor the chest with its foreboding saw-requiring thoracic cavity so close under the surface.

Eventually, a few days in, once your own nerves are out of the way, you'll flip your new friend sunny-side-up to hide the clumsy early mistakes of your rookie hands and have a fresh start — when revealing the heart won't feel so personal and tender, when the face will seem like nothing more than twelve cranial nerves covered inconveniently by slowly rotting flesh, after the brutish cataloging of increasingly minute body parts has rendered a former human being into exactly the sum of its parts and nothing more.

Take mind of this feeling.

You will need it.

CHAPTER 1

Every earthquake starts with a moment of disbelief. How could it not? When previously firm ground suddenly reveals itself to be a formless liquid wave, who among us would not start by concluding they are dreaming?

Dr. Maggie Owens was looking up at the ceiling when she felt the first tremble. It was subtle, just a minor shift of her feet, a tilt of the window, a brief disorientation, just enough to send her hands out to her sides, searching for walls but grasping only air. The sensation passed. Her stance widened, and she looked down at the now-still ground accusingly. Had it really moved? *It must have been nothing.* She brought her eyes back up to the ceiling.

The vaulted atrium in which she stood was on the top floor of the tallest building in the sprawling complex that made up Portland University Hospital; a hospital compound situated at the edge of a precipice just south of downtown. The hospital, once built so high on this hill to separate the infirm from the healthy people of a good society, had recently decided to lean into its viewpoint status and become not just a place of healing, but a tourist destination of sorts. As such, the atrium featured a city-themed gift shop, high end coffee, and a milieu of people along the entire spectrum from calamity to recreation — grieving families searching for meaning in the panoramic mountain view, spent hospital workers escaping the grind, new parents wondering what the hell they'd just got into, interloping tourists snapping photos of the riverfront below while drinking six dollar coffees and planning their river cruise.

In the center, Maggie examined the curves of a blown-glass sculpture that dangled overhead, a spectacular centerpiece suspended by cables from the ceiling. The piece was an octopodian wonder, swirls of colored tentacles jutting out in every direction like a dare, casting prisms of green and blue light upon the polished floor. In the early-morning light, the rising of the sun sent the reflections into undulating waves on the floor.

Like an aquarium, thought Maggie, *and I am the fish.*

As she looked on, she noted the slightest hint of sway to the sculpture, which seemed to be pulling at its cable attachments on one side, releasing fine dust to the ground below. *That's weird,* Maggie thought, as a wave of vertigo passed over her and forced her to sit down on the bench beside her. Maggie startled as a *clang* rang out from the coffee shop; a barista had dropped the pitcher from her milk steamer onto the hard floor. Maggie gripped the bench harder and pressed her feet into the floor.

Wait, is this bench moving too?

Yes. Yes, the bench was moving, and the floor too, in a sine wave that now had countless other items careening around the hard linoleum in a cacophonous symphony. *This isn't real,* thought Maggie. *This isn't real.* She closed her eyes tightly as her vision started to tunnel, and a loud ringing took over her hearing. Through this static she heard a voice call out behind, or beside, (or above) her: "Earthquake! Stop, drop and roll, everybody!"

Wrong catchphrase, Maggie thought, *but close enough.* She held on tighter, peeking an eye open to try to judge whether she could reasonably get her body to shelter underneath the bench. On the floor, the rainbow reflections of that diabolical glass sculpture were now swirling in mad, frantic patterns at her feet. *How long could this go on until the cables give out,* she thought, *and the angry tentacles come crashing down to impale me?*

Maggie put her head down and covered her neck with her hands, back curved up as an offering, waiting for the certainty of something terrible. Even in her readiness, her body still startled as something did come down upon her shoulder. It wasn't glass, though; it was too soft a touch. A tap, actually. It tapped again.

"Ma'am? Are you okay? Are you okay?"

The voice and the hand seemed to steady not just Maggie but the ground itself, and everything returned to stillness.

"Ma'am?"

Maggie let her breath out and turned her head up to find a young man in a short white coat crouching beside her. He had a hand on her shoulder and kind brown eyes. Maggie took another deep breath and looked a little higher. The sculpture was motionless, secure, intact. The tourists were standing and snapping their photos. The espresso machine whirred on, making coffee. She blinked.

"Yeah, I — sorry. I have a little vertigo at height, I guess," she said. A lie, but one without consequence, right?

The young man patted her shoulder in understanding. "Try looking out into the distance, instead of down," he said. "It'll help."

Maggie straightened the rest of the way up on the bench, thanked the young man, and sent him away.

This isn't real.

Maggie's therapist called these little incidents *flashbacks,* which didn't feel quite right, but Maggie had no other word to identify them. Visions? Alternate realities? Whatever they were, she'd been having them periodically over the last year, often triggered by a sudden loud noise in a crowd. Mostly, they passed quickly and without consequence. It was unnerving to have been clocked by a bystander, a medical student no less. She'd have to try harder to keep it together. She looked out into the distance, as recommended, trying to enjoy the view.

It had been a year since Maggie had last stepped foot in any hospital, and ten years since she'd last been in this one. She'd thought it would feel like a homecoming. *It's the perfect setup,* she had told Joan, her therapist, requesting clearance to start working again. *Work will be therapeutic,* Maggie had said, *to have a purpose again.* Now, Maggie hoped she wouldn't embarrass them both.

What are five things you can see? Joan asked in Maggie's head as she looked out into the distance. A river cut a gentle scar through the city in the middle distance, carrying mud and feces and fentanyl from the inlands to the Oregon coast. Beyond that, just at the horizon, Maggie could just make out the blown top of Mt. St. Helen's through the clouds, a reminder perhaps, or a warning.

A hawk circled outside the window, looking for its next meal within the thicket of trees that cascaded down the hillside, encircling the hospital complex on all sides. Even as the sprawl of the city had since commercialized everything else for a hundred miles, this patch of wildness had remained untouched around the perimeter. Crossing over this natural boundary, a set of thick cables pulled a glass and silver aerial tram car up from the riverfront, moving people from the abundant parking on the industrial riverfront up to the hospital. The car swung gently in the wind, and Maggie felt the floor move again. She looked out at the mountain with accusation.

What are four things you can feel? Joan insisted on knowing. Does nausea count? The sweat on her palms? The urge to urinate? As she searched for a fourth feeling, her watch buzzed with a notification, graciously fulfilling the quota.

Orientation, the watch advised, was occurring in one hour. Thankful for the reminder of work to ground her, Maggie abandoned Joan's voice in favor of her phone. She swiped it open and clicked on an icon labeled *p*Value,* inside the outline of an anatomically correct human heart.

A tag line flashed on the screen: *Build up some STEAM in your love life,* which was then replaced with the image of a shirtless man. He stood holding a dead fish, smiling proudly.

Joe, the caption said below the photo. *43. Pathologist, Musician, World Citizen, Animal Lover.*

Maggie swiped left. A woman appeared.

Suzanne, 39. Neuroscience Post-Doctorate by day, Musician at night. Just holding on to this blue marble like everyone else. She is somehow also holding a fish. The fish is dead.

Maggie swiped left again. She sighed and looked out the window, just in time to watch as a gust of wind sent the cabled tram car into an elliptical sway on the way up to its perch. Her palms began to sweat again in sympathy for the car's occupants. She clenched and unclenched her fists, trying to focus on the feeling of relaxation. *These hands have broken ribs,* she said to the car in her mind. The car didn't seem to notice her bravado.

What are three things you can hear? Joan insisted on knowing, but Maggie swiped her away and turned back to *p*Value*.

Brad, 45, Doctor of Physical Therapy. Would love to build up some dynamic tension with you. Picture of him, mostly muscles, dangling off the side of a rock wall. She swiped left again. The tram car continued to wind up and up, until it was an unavoidable presence in her field of vision. She fought the urge to look away. *Avoidance amplifies fear,* Joan would have said. *Avoidance is your enemy.*

So she looked. She may as well face the reality that she would be working so high above sea level, so reliant on the skill and diligence of building engineers, no matter her mode of transport.

The cables certainly seemed sturdy (Maggie told herself), and were designed by engineers (she reasoned), and were governed by the laws of physics (in which she believed, as a scientist herself), and were regulated by building codes (which still existed, even in these chaotic times). The building codes would keep them all safe, wouldn't they?

Building codes are written in blood, she thought, before she could stop herself. She'd heard this saying recently on a news report about a collapsed condominium building in Florida. Her mind moved on to the next obvious questions: *What building codes have yet to be written? And in whose blood?* Most people in that building had been sleeping during the collapse, blissfully unaware they were about to write a building code. *Whose blood? Could it be mine?*

With that in mind, Maggie leaned forward and rested her forehead on the glass, staring down the sheer cliff and leaning into the feeling of tingling and weakening legs. A few pops of color peeked through the trees below, marking the presence of tents for the unhoused that were being erected and swept in cycles around the city. The tents had no answer for her, except to say that her problems were minuscule in comparison to the scale of human suffering, so what did it matter anyhow?

On the far side of the river, the remnants of an overnight fire smoldered, flanked by a single fire truck. The fire (she would learn later on the city subreddit) had taken out an abandoned bookstore and all its abandoned books, leaving only a cauterized patch of carbon in its place. The conflagration had seemingly consumed the building entirely in one gulp before burning itself out, leaving the surrounding foliage unharmed.

Maggie had an idea.

She turned to stand with her back to the window and snapped a selfie with the fire truck and the smoldering rubble in the background. She chose *Al Power* out of her contacts and sent the photo with the caption: *Burning Man's gonna burn, amirite?* She put the phone back in her pocket and stared out across the water.

Maggie did not yet know what she would know later about Al. This is the state we are all in, of course, at all times, the not knowing now what we will know later. Fully enveloped in the bliss of not knowing, Maggie smiled the secret smile of ignorance as she eyed the scene of last night's crime from a safe distance and contemplated the motives of the Burning Man.

The Burning Man was a name locals had given to a community arsonist who'd been prolific that summer, burning away small clearings in the city's growing slime mold of public garbage almost every night. He wasn't officially publicly sanctioned, of course, but he may as well have been. Most of what burned was unwanted, and the fires were met mostly with relief. The fire department had put out various statements on the matter, stood up a hotline, made waves in the local news, but it was half-hearted at best. Someone must have been responsible for it. The surface wasn't quite hot enough yet to invoke spontaneous combustion, not here anyhow. When no specific someone could be identified, The Burning Man had been born into the public imagination of online forums. There was a palpable collective resignation in the comments: *If the city isn't going to take care of this garbage, at least someone will.* Certain vocal people felt he was doing the city a favor, for which it should be thankful, as the fires had scuttled many unhoused folks out of the city in search of better air quality. *And maybe what we need isn't more housing, but fewer people.*

The Burning Man was in this way the city's own Batman, if the bat signal were trash, and the Joker were trash, and Poison Ivy were trash, and the Batmobile only spit fire on everything to turn it to ash. A twenty-first-century alchemist, using old magic to turn the items into something bigger than themselves. All better off for their flight into the already-doomed atmosphere, somehow.

Maggie could relate with the sentiment.

As she contemplated the fire, Maggie sat back on the bench and ran a hand through her long brown ponytail, absent-mindedly pulling her hair around to her nose for a sniff. It smelled of tobacco from her morning cigarette, an indulgence she had reintroduced last year in her own fit of nihilism. *What's the use when I'll probably die in a great flood before I ever get emphysema?* Still, she recoiled at the odor and set her phone down into her lap, rustling around in the bag for a small bottle of hospital-grade deodorizing spray, which gave a fine mist to her ponytail and shirt collar.

Just as she was smelling her fingers, her wristwatch buzzed again. A reply from Al? No, just Christopher.

Hey Babe. Was just thinking about you this morning. Hope your first day goes well.

Pause. She let out a tiny groan that echoed back against the glass, causing her to instinctively check over her shoulder to see who might have heard it. An older woman sat three chairs down, holding a tissue to her mouth silently. She paid no mind to Maggie.

Reply? At that moment, the now-descending silver tram car caught just the right prismatic angle of morning light to reflect a focused beam directly into her pupils, causing her to squint and look away. A message, she thought, from the universe. She had left Missouri for a reason. She was here now, sitting in this West Coast eagle's nest, deliberately hundreds of miles away.

She swiped the message away and tapped again on the logo for *p*Value.*

Billie, 37. Chiropractic student, cat owner, home brewer. I'm a high velocity, low amplitude kinda gal, but the frequency is up to you. Picture of her lying in bed, seemingly shirtless, a long-haired, brown tabby draped across her chest. Pause. *What would Al do?* Pause. Swipe right. *Maybe Al already has.*

As if timed to the swipe, at that moment a voice from somewhere started singing quietly in time with the overhead muzak, and Maggie wrinkled her nose and looked over at the woman with the tissue, who was looking sideways back at her as the voice echoed through the atrium. It only took a moment longer for Maggie to realize where the song was coming from. It was a song meant just for her.

"Frankieeeee, Fraaaaaankie, he's a man with a plaaaaan. He ain't got skin but he's got two hands, and he'll never be lonely agaaaaaaain," the voice sang.

A woman peeked her head over Maggie's shoulder with a wide Cheshire grin. She had dark hair pulled taut into a ballet bun and mahogany eyes that made wide, intent eye contact. Her white coat gleamed with a bleached intensity; both the coat and her skin were immaculate. *Dr. J. Oliver,* read the embroidery on her coat, *Department of Dermatology*. She had a black surgical mask pulled below her chin.

"Maggie Oooooooowens," sang the woman in faux-operatic vibrato at the conclusion of her little performance, opening her arms to signal an intention to hug. "Can't hide from *me,* girlie. I saw your reflection in the glass. What the heck are you doing back at the *PUH?*" This was pronounced with a long *ooo* sound, like *poo.* "I thought you were in, like, Kansas or something?"

This was the danger of returning to an old haunt; the ghosts there will remember you. Maggie stood to greet the woman, who was already coming in for a hug. Maggie leaned back reflexively, her arms moving up, then down, then up again as she tried to configure her body appropriately to receive the greeting.

"Jess Oliver, in the flesh. I was hoping you'd still be here," Maggie said, patting Jess on the shoulder and pulling herself away. Jess had been in Maggie's Gross Anatomy lab group in medical school, and was the very first person Maggie had ever met here, in fact. Fitting she'd be the first to greet her on her prodigal return.

Jess grabbed Maggie by the arms and looked her up and down.

"What has it been, ten years since graduation?"

"Almost to the day, I think." Maggie pulled an arm free to hide the phone and its *p*Value* secrets in her bag.

"You missed the reunion," Jess said, frowning. She lowered her voice, adding, "You know everyone was really worried, right? We *heard* that you and Christoper were at —"

"Oh, yeah, I'd rather not — " Maggie rubbed her palms on her pants and looked down.

"— *Jackson County Memorial*," Jess said in a hushed tone, not taking the hint. "Were you there for, well, you know, the *shooting?*" The last word was swallowed into a whisper, as if it would conjure a bad spirit to say it aloud.

Maggie nodded and looked at her feet.

"You were *there?* Like, *during* — " Jess' eyes were wide, and she gripped Maggie's upper arm.

"Yeah, I-I'm fine, though. Really! Intact. See? No bullet holes!" Maggie patted her body down to emphasize the point.

The two paused in a silent, involuntary remembrance for a moment, and Jess hugged her again. This time Maggie allowed it, imagining Joan watching proudly from across the room.

"Jess," Maggie interrupted, wanting to change the subject. "Isn't this a little early in the morning for a dermatologist?" She glanced at her watch, which read 6:45 AM.

Jess gave her an eye roll and looked around with a *don't ask* look. "Yes, it *is* too early for a dermatologist, way too early for the *Chief* of Dermatology, if you ask me, but here I am."

"Of course, of *course* you are. Congratulations. So, what is the *Chief* of Dermatology doing up so early?"

Jess glanced behind her shoulder at the well-dressed receptionist sitting attentively at her desk, at the tissue-holding woman who was now staring at them, and at the echo chamber of glass windows and high ceilings that surrounded them. She frowned.

"Right now, I'm headed to the Doctor's Lounge for some coffee. Take the stairs down with me?"

This was stated as a question, but Jess already had her hand on Maggie's elbow in such a way as to lead her toward the stairwell. Maggie followed without resistance, taking one last suspicious look up at the swirling glass of the Chihuly sculpture as she passed under it. As they ducked into the stairwell, the glass and shine and din of the lobby gave way to concrete and quiet, like stepping backstage in a theater mid-performance.

Jess stopped to take off her heels for the trip down. "Good God, I wish it weren't my job to look so damn *good* all the time. Beauty is pain, you know?"

"I guess that's the job, right?" Maggie stood wearing her worn Danskos, plain face, and basic ponytail. "I mean, as the *Chief* of Dermatology."

Jess was proceeding down the stairs in her stockinged feet, holding her shoes slung casually in one hand, craning her neck backwards to look at Maggie as they chatted and descended. Maggie held tight to the railing, prepared to catch Jess by the arm if need be.

"Let me just *tell you* about this morning," Jess was saying. "Some VIP donor had a hip replacement yesterday — god *forbid* he got a little contact dermatitis from the chlorhexidine skin prep. *Big* emergency, *very* serious, of course. So *of course* it was necessary for the *Chief* of Dermatology to *personally* come apply the cortisol to his *poor wittle scrotum* before starting clinic today."

"Hope you laid it on thick. Mama needs her signing bonus, right?"

Jess laughed, feet gliding frictionlessly down the stairs. "Whatever keeps the water flowing," she said. "Wait, *signing* bonus? Does that mean you're back here? Like, *back* here?"

"Yeah, I'll be rounding with the internal medicine residents." Maggie tried to sound happy about it. "Back to my roots."

Jess smiled a plastic smile. "Oh, what fun!"

Maggie shrugged. "Can't be worse than county hospital life, you know? What with — well, seems like you heard. Dr. March is still the Chief of Medicine, so, you know. He took pity on me, I think."

"Took pity, my ass! I'll bet March can't believe his luck to get you back here. And all it took was, um, well. . ." Jess paused, clearing her throat, not finishing the thought. "Anyway! That's great news. *Great* news. I've missed you."

The two walked a bit longer in silence, Jess in her soft and silent feet, Maggie plodding loudly in her Danskos. A few floors down, Jess broke the silence again.

"You know, you could've called? After, well, *you know*. The *thing*. Everyone thought you and Christopher were *dead* because we didn't hear from you."

Jess said the word *dead* in a forced whisper that echoed around the concrete stairwell. They passed Floor 7 and Maggie was starting to feel slightly out of breath, so she tried to subtly slow their pace as well as change the subject.

"Well, funny you should say that," Maggie started, taking a deep breath and pausing mid-thought. Before she could continue, Jess gasped and stopped walking abruptly, causing Maggie to nearly bowl her over from behind. Maggie ended up catching herself on the railing, but not before falling out of her shoes. She was trying to gather herself and apologize to Jess, who in return was falling over herself to apologize back to Maggie.

"NO, oh shit, *shit!* I'm sorry, don't tell me he's actually, *actually,* um, *you know —*"

"Dead?" Maggie realized her error. "No! Oh, noooo, no no no, *he's* not dead, oh gosh, yeah I can see how you would, um, well." Maggie caught herself, taking a deep breath to reset. "It's just that *we* are. . .well, you know." Maggie couldn't get herself to say the word, so she held up her empty ring finger instead. Jess groaned and pouted her lower lip exaggeratedly.

"You too? Damn." Jess held up her own empty ring finger. "Guess that's going around. Was it because of — gosh, I don't know how to say it — did you break up because of. . .because of, well." Jess stopped there. A dermatologist does not have to contend with tragedy, thought Maggie, in forgiveness. Not like an internist.

"Oh, you know Christopher. He was exactly the hero they deserved, you know? He needed to stay, I needed to leave."

"Well! His loss is our gain," Jess said, trying to find something to be cheerful for. "I'm just glad to hear you're both alive, I was convinced that Frank had maybe cursed our lab group forever. Like, *Final Destination* or something. You know that movie?"

"Jess, that's preposterous. Not that I even believe in curses, but *Frank* would never. Never! I'll bet we're the closest thing he ever had to family."

"Either way, I'm relieved to know I'm not the last one standing, that's all." Jess turned around and gave Maggie a little wink, as she added, "I thought about calling you, but I was afraid to know. You're a real asshole for not calling." Jess stopped and turned around to emphasize her point. "At least post something on the SocialEyes group or *something,*" she said, referring to the social media site their medical school class had used to keep in touch.

"Ha! Didn't you hear SocialEyes is bad for mental health? We were all supposed to delete it."

"Maggie."

"I know, I know. But look, we're here now, aren't we? Alive and well! Well, alive at least."

Maggie had missed a clue here. Maggie will soon know she needs to look for clues, study the details of language, take nothing for granted, but she didn't yet know this. Maggie didn't yet know she should think like a detective. The moment passed.

"Are we, though?" Jess wondered as she slipped her shoes back on and opened the door for Maggie to walk through. As Maggie started to pass, Jess became momentarily distracted, turning up a wrinkled nose to say, "Whoa. Whoa! Why do you smell like bathroom spray?"

Maggie shrugged, averted her eyes, and tried to continue.

"Maggie!" Jess barred the door with an arm and put on her best stern mother voice. "You're not *smoking* again, are you? I thought you gave that shit up!"

Maggie blushed. Her breathing shallowed and her heart rate went up as the accusation hit her, the same physical response one might have to a first kiss, a Vodka Red Bull, a bungee jump, a thrill ride. This was the score her body was keeping, and the shame was the point.

"I don't know what you're talking about, Jess," Maggie said with that tone people use when they aren't really trying to hide the lie.

"Girl, you *know* how much hell that habit will bring upon your skin, right? You gotta think about these things now that you're *single.*"

"Ugh, dating is the *last* thing on my mind right now," Maggie said, convincingly. As she said this, her watch buzzed with a notification from *p*Value. You passed the t-test,* the watch said, *It's a match!* Maggie put her hand in her pocket to hide it from view.

The two women spilled out of the stairwell, back on stage, into the chaotic morning foot traffic. Jess kept a quick pace as they weaved through tottering patients and towering surgeons, down the wide halls of the main arterial.

"Look familiar?" Jess craned her head back to give Maggie a wink.

"No, actually," Maggie answered, guiding Jess gently with one hand as she barely avoided bowling over a pregnant woman who had stopped to take a breath ahead of them. "Everything looks completely different."

These halls were the same halls her feet had worn thin during her four years as a medical student. However, in the time since she'd left, the halls had been subject to the smoothing forces of capitalism and modern design, forces that had come to splash faux-hardwood laminate, matte tile accents, and soft-hued lighting onto every inner surface. Off-white walls had been replaced with high-definition photo murals, marketing the promise of happy, thriving faces leaping across grassy fields. Hallways leading to Obstetrics were emblazoned with cherubic model-baby faces cradled by nurturing and diverse model-mothers and model-fathers. Pathways to the ICU were lined with weathered old hands cradled in the grasp of smoother young hands, presumably saying a silent goodbye.

"Just wait until you see the hallway to Human Resources," Jess said with another wink.

"Why?"

Jess started to answer, but then stopped abruptly in front of a heavy wooden door. "Oh! Here we are." A worn brass plaque on the door identified their destination. "This is where the magic happens."

"Doctor's Lounge" was actually a misnomer, as the door now opened for a wide set of non-physician credentials (NP, PA, CNM, CRNA, et cetera, a list that grew year-over-year); there had been a suggestion at some point to make it a "Provider's Lounge," but no one really gave a shit to fight *for* this change, so the few who gave many shits to fight *against* it won out, and the anachronistic name stood fast at the threshold, a testament to the stickiness of old hierarchies. Lounge, too, was not entirely accurate; like many spaces in the remote-work era, the lounge had slowly been infiltrated by decidedly non-lounge pursuits. First, by laptops and pocket phones that pulled at their owners' leashes, then eventually by formalized workstations that lined the walls, and now, a separate auxiliary workroom in the back filled with more workstations. The lounge was no longer so much an escape from work as a rebranding of it, like WeWork had opened up a co-working space at your actual place of business.

Jess pulled Maggie into a line for the coffee carafes, and Maggie pulled out her phone instinctively as they waited.

The phone seemed to know she was in a hospital. On her social feeds, posts about pets and babies in Missouri were intermingled with ads for drugs with unpronounceable names like Wybnasta and Ryverbi and Vrabnallix. *Keep life moving,* said an advertisement for a monoclonal constipation remedy. *Clear your schedule and your skin for life*, said an advertisement for a non-steroidal eczema cream. *Focus on what's important,* with this new isomer for ADHD. Maggie paused her scroll at an ad for Strizyndi, a new oral glucagon analog. *Jump start your journey to health*, it said. Her thumb hovered over it for a moment, considering.

"Oh, thank *god,*" Jess turned around to say before Maggie could double tap. "Looks like they brought back the donuts. *Jesus Christ,* I thought I might have to riot."

Maggie looked up, feeling the stretchy waist line of her slacks acutely. "They got rid of donuts?"

"Yeah, some jerk-off admin on the Wellness Committee thought they should take all the concentrated sugar out of the hospital, *as if.*"

They finally got to the front of the line, where Jess carefully cut a

15-degree triangle out of a plain cake donut and filled up a black coffee before ducking back out into the crowd. Maggie grabbed an apple fritter and a half-caff and turned around to find Jess gone. *Some people never change,* she thought.

The room was larger than she'd anticipated but still looked crowded as folks formed tight bubbles around the tables like a high school cafeteria. In one corner, square-jawed orthopedic surgeons discussed the finer points of mountain biking, and in another, sunken-eyed post-call obstetricians and midwives compared shoe inserts. Along the far wall, a table of wild-haired neurologists regarded each other through spectacles that were either laughably too small or too large for their faces. In the coffee line, with no time to sit, critical care docs rolled through with a knowing swagger before rolling right out again. There was an order to things here. You didn't have to fit into these stereotypes, but it certainly helped if you did.

Maggie was looking for Jess, but if she was to be truly honest with herself (which she almost never was), she was also looking for someone else. She was starting to give up when a friendly call came from across the fray, and her hair stood on end for just a second.

"Hey, is that Maggie OWENS? Class of 2015?"

This was not Jess' voice, but it was familiar. She searched for its owner.

"Over here," the voice said again.

It was the baritone voice of a man, who was standing up and waving to Maggie from a table full of what Maggie had to assume were surgeons, lean and muscled young people chowing down on plates piled high with bacon and drinking from comically sized bottles that probably held some kind of proteinaceous fitness goo. Maggie caught the man's eye and pushed her way over to the table, spilling only a small dollop of coffee on her pant leg as she did so.

"If it isn't Marcus Pelletier, male model and kick-ass surgeon," Maggie said as she approached.

Maggie's reference to his modeling career came from the fact that in school, Marcus' face had graced nearly every brochure, web page, email, and tour guide put out by the school's marketing department.

No doubt this was in part because he was an attractive guy with a wide, inviting smile. However, the marketing department's interest in him may have had more to do with his status as a black student in this supposedly liberal, but still very monochromatic school.

Marcus made a face at the *male model* reference, and Maggie immediately regretted having made it. She tried to make up for it with a congenial side hug, which Marcus accepted. Though he'd put on a few pounds (as they all had), he was still firmly on the attractive side of dad bod. Maggie noted the absence of any gold band on his finger; a habit she had recently and reluctantly picked up.

"Maggie, I *heard* you were coming back," Marcus said, breaking their hug with a percussive slap on the back. "But I barely believed it. It's been too long!"

"Word travels fast, I guess." Maggie hadn't exactly announced her return, but a hospital is a closed system — new information has nowhere to go but everywhere. Marcus turned to the table of residents who were stuffing their faces and engaging in some kind of heated debate about suture preferences.

"Dr. Owens here was top of our class," Marcus told the surgical residents, who were in no way paying attention to Maggie's arrival; the comment had not been for their benefit, anyhow. Maggie shook her head and smiled.

"If I remember correctly, *you* beat *me* out in the class rankings."

"And would you look at us both, right back here in *this* shithole."

"But what a *golden* shithole it is these days," Maggie responded, and Marcus laughed generously. Maggie recalled Marcus had stayed here, in this mid-tier hospital, despite the potential to match anywhere he wanted for residency, due to concerns for an ailing grandmother, a disabled sibling, and other *real-life shit*.

"For now, anyhow. Sit down and catch up," Marcus said. "My first case is still getting prepped."

Maggie sat down and started with the standard catch-up talk; was he married, how old are the kids, what are they doing, do you still talk to *x* or *y* classmate. Marcus was divorced, but had two kids, five and eight.

"What about you, though? You and Christopher have any yet?"

Marcus had kind, competent eyes and an earnest face as he asked this, a face to convince a person he had just met that he ought to cut their body open while they sleep. Still, even to this face, Maggie had a hard time saying it.

"Well, Christopher and I . . ." She drifted off, losing the words. She again pointed to her empty ring finger, wondering how many times she would repeat this move before the end of the day.

"Damn, you too," Marcus said, lowering his voice. "Sorry to hear. Maybe I shouldn't have pried."

"No, no, it's fine, it's fine. Luckily no kids, though. Just two sad adults. So, you know." She took a deep breath. "I guess that's going around, huh?"

"Is that why you came back here, then?"

"Well," Maggie said, "there was more to it, I suppose." Maggie looked over at the residents at the table, who were now comparing nearby rock-climbing routes, definitely not interested in Maggie's life story. She spoke softly anyhow. "I was in Missouri, you know. At Jackson County Memorial? Before. When. Um. . ." She trailed off, looking at Marcus' face to see if he recognized her meaning. Marcus gasped.

"Oh, shit, that's right! Were you —were you *there*? Like, *there* there?" Marcus was gripping Maggie's forearm on the table while he said this.

"Yeah. Yeah, I was there. *There* there." Maggie cast her eyes down at her shoes. "So, you know. I was off work for a while, thought I'd get a fresh start somewhere familiar."

"Oh, jeez. Fuck, dammit Mags. Was Christopher —"

"Oh, no, no, he's just fine. He was at home when it happened. Luckily, I guess. He probably would have jumped into the line of fire if he'd had the chance."

"*Damn.*"

"So, you know. I heard through the grapevine they were offering full loan repayment as a sign-on here, and the *salary*, well, you know. Hard to turn down. I guess that was as good a reason as any. Turns out a girl has a price." Maggie shrugged.

Had Maggie sold out? Perhaps, yes. Technically. Maggie is a fish, though, and the system is an ocean which has consumed all dry land, and her only skill is to swim. So what?

"Don't we all!" Marcus said, trying to lighten the mood. "Funny how a 30 billion dollar windfall to the hospital endowment suddenly means we're fully staffed. *Everybody* has a price, Mags."

"Yes, well. Not *everyone*. Not Christopher." She shrugged. "He got an offer too, but he felt an obligation to stay put. 'Didn't want to abandon the troops' or something. Never mind *me*, of course. So. . ." Maggie's voice trailed off. "Well! I guess you're all caught up?" Maggie gave another apologetic shrug. "Sorry to hit you with all that."

Was this oversharing? Perhaps by normal workplace standards. But what was oversharing with a person who once stood next to you holding the same retractor in a six-hour bowel resection surgery? What was oversharing with a person who later warned you to change your scrubs because you had a little blood soaking through the crotch? With a person who has seen you cry silently while trying to operate the camera in a gallbladder case, during which an elder surgeon is yelling at you to get the cystic duct into view, a structure that you quite frankly never learned to locate and never will?

Marcus let out a long sigh. "Well, shit. I guess I'm glad to have you back, regardless. Finally get some brain power back around here." Marcus gave a pointed look as he said this. Maggie laughed in that nervous way that people laugh at a compliment, if that's what this was.

"It's fun to be here, anyhow. Like going back to high school or something, wondering who I'm going to run into." Maggie was surveying the crowd, subtly she hoped, as she said this. "Maybe I should just send out a bulk email letting everyone know at once, so I don't have to keep telling the story over and over. Christopher and I deleted our SocialEyes accounts seven years ago, so we can't just like, *change our status* like the kids are doing these days."

"SocialEyes?" Marcus laughed. "Maggie, the kids aren't using *SocialEyes* anymore. Only us oldheads use SocialEyes. You should make an account, though, get back on the class page. It's mostly a dumpster fire, but there are some advantages." Marcus lowered his voice again. "Keeping tabs on who's single, for one," he said with a wink. "Not to mention *dead, you know what I mean?*"

Marcus was shaking his head in that way that said, *but what're you gonna do, right?* Maggie continued laughing out of reflex until she clocked what Marcus had said and her laughter attenuated and then stopped. She went through some quick math in her head, measuring out the emotional cost of knowing the information versus the cost of not knowing the information; math that was hard to do without knowing the actual weight of the components. Marcus' eyes grew wider with alarm as he realized she did not, in fact, know what he meant.

Maggie was startled out of her mental arithmetic by a hand on her shoulder. She spun to see Jess standing above her.

"What's up, Marcus? Did you see what the *cash* dragged home?" Jess was proud of her little pun and was about to slug Maggie jokingly on the shoulder when she clocked the dour expression on Marcus' face and the furrowing of Maggie's brow. "Dude, why the serious faces? Did somebody die or what?"

"Yeah, that's the question. Did someone die?"

Marcus sighed. "She's not on SocialEyes, Jess."

"Oh, SHIT. Like, you didn't know about, well, *you know.*"

"No Jess, I don't know what you're talking about."

Jess began to stutter, taking a step back from Maggie. "Not even, you know? Not even, right? I mean, I just assumed you *knew* — I mean, because you guys, well, you had a — right? You know?"

Maggie put her hand on Jess' arm to stop her. "Jess, I *don't know* who you're talking about."

Jess pulled a chair over and sat next to Maggie, looking her pointedly in the eyes and pausing for a second. "Well, OK. Are you sure you want to know all this?" Jess' hand was on her pager, and her eyes began to dart not-too-subtly to the door. "I mean, you've already been through so much, right?"

Maggie smiled an unnaturally wide *I'm fine* smile, saying, "Whatever it is, I'll be fine."

Jess paused for what seemed like a full minute, trying to parse Maggie's face as if to gauge it for some feature that would reassure her.

She finally broke her silence. "Okay, then. Okay. Okay." Jess looked at Marcus, who looked back at Jess. Maggie was looking at them both.

"Okay guys, out with it," Maggie said. "Anyone I know?" Maggie's tone clearly relayed an assumption that it was not anyone she knew, or at least not anyone she felt would deal an emotional blow of any kind.

Building codes are written in blood. The rebar was beginning to bend and sway, and the outer shell of masonry was beginning to crumble off the side of the building, and Maggie was still in a deep slumber. The memory of her last cigarette would soon feel distant and small, and would not be there to soften the landing.

"C'mon, guys," Maggie said to the piteous, reluctant faces of Jess and Marcus. "There is *literally nothing* you can tell me that can top what I've been through this year. Just get out with it already."

Maggie felt confident in this statement when she made it, the type of confidence a building inspector may have used when declaring a Florida condo building safe for habitation.

Was it really the inspector's fault, though? Wasn't that building doomed from the start? When they built it using that too-soft stone, so close to the too-salty ocean and its too-harsh winds? When they filled it full of people who wrongly assumed the building codes would keep them safe? People who had forgotten that building codes are written in blood, and that their bodies are full of just this type of ink?

"Maggie, you aren't going to like it," Jess said.

Maggie cocked her head sideways and frowned. "Hit me, Jess. I am *invincible* with therapy right now."

Jess shrugged and started in.

"Well, first of all, I guess we don't actually know *for sure* what happened. Right, Marcus? We don't know for *sure*." A dermatologist does not know how to talk about death. Not like a surgeon or an internist.

Maggie frowned. "We don't know *what* for sure, Jess? And about *who?*"

Jess closed her eyes to not see the aftermath.

"Alice? The news is about *Alice.*"

"Alice who?" Maggie was searching her internal Rolodex of classmates to place the person, realizing that no fewer than four different Alices could be the one in question. She started with the one she knew the least. "Pediatrics Alice?"

"No, Maggie." Maggie was falling, but she didn't yet know it.

"Neuro Alice?"

"*No*, Maggie."

"Other Neuro Alice?"

"Maggie." Jess was boring her eyes into Maggie's with an uncomfortable intensity while nodding her head slowly up and down, willing Maggie to come up with the answer so she wouldn't have to say it.

"Maggie," she said. "Maggie." More nodding. "*MAGGIE.*"

The rebar had snapped in two with a loud *thwap*, and Maggie was now awakened to the feeling of falling. A building code was about to be written.

"MAGGIE." Repeating Maggie's name was all Jess could seem to muster, but it gave Maggie the information she required. As Jess continued to nod and repeat, nod and repeat, Maggie slowly started shaking her head.

"No," she said.

"Yes," Jess said in return.

"NO!"

Jess was silent this time.

"Not *my* Alice? Al? *Al?* Al. Al Power? She can't be, I just — wait, did you say you're not sure of something?" Maggie was now looking accusatorially at Jess, the messenger in the line of fire.

Marcus piped in. "Jess, we're sure. I'm sure, anyway. Don't sugarcoat it."

"Sugarcoat *what?*" Maggie looked at Marcus, then Jess, then back at Marcus, who was giving Maggie a suspicious side-eye.

"Weren't you guys, like, thick as thieves? How is it possible you don't know any of this? It was all over the SocialEyes group, anyhow."

Maggie had the start of a tear welling up in just one eye, but she suppressed it.

"SocialEyes? SocialEyes? We were all *supposed* to delete it, remember?"

Jess shook her head and said in a small voice, "I can't believe you don't know *anything,* though. Didn't you guys talk all the time?"

"We were — we had — *that's not the point,*" Maggie stammered. "So what happened?"

Marcus looked side-eyed over at the group of residents, and Jess spoke in hushed tones that made Maggie lean in with one ear forward. Jess cleared her throat and looked at Marcus, who cleared his throat and looked back at her. Neither wanting to take full responsibility, they volleyed the story back and forth between them in fits and starts.

"Well, it started with a surgical complication," Jess started, before looking at Marcus and pausing. "Marcus might know more about that."

"Yeah, your girl *fell asleep* in a lap chole," Marcus said, referring to the laparoscopic removal of a gallbladder, the most routine of all general surgeries. "Passed right the fuck out, face-first onto the sterile field. Severed the splenic artery in the process." Maggie gasped out loud. Even as an internist, she knew a splenic artery laceration to be a hilariously bad misadventure during a gallbladder removal.

"Was she post-call or something?"

"Nah, Maggie. She was *drunk,*" Marcus said. "The patient was eventually fine, *thank god,* but you can imagine how risk management felt about it."

"When did this happen?"

Marcus looked over at Jess, who picked up the thread.

"Maybe six months ago?"

Maggie noticed an acrid smell creeping into the room as Jess continued, which she tried to swat away with disbelief. *Was this a dream?* she thought. *This must be a dream.*

Jess was continuing on. "Her license got suspended, obviously. She was in that, that — what do you call it?" Jess looked now at Marcus for help.

"Wellness Program, I think," Marcus said.

"Yeah! That's it, Wellness Program. Weird name for it, but that's the one where you can get your license back by getting drug tested and stuff? She did that for a while, seemed like she might come back from it. But then she kind of, well. Relapsed, maybe?"

Maggie's nose was recoiling now at the smell, which was overpowering her ability to ignore it. She put a hand up over her mouth to breathe through the sleeve of her fleece pullover.

Jess noticed and paused her storytelling. "Are you okay? Should I continue?"

"Do you, um, smell something?"

Jess shook her head. "Just coffee and donuts. Are you sure you want to hear this?"

Maggie motioned her to continue, her eyes now watering.

"At one point, Al posted this weird video on SocialEyes. She had shaved her head, and was talking about being a fisherman. She seemed, well, kinda wasted."

A fisherman.

Jess stopped there and looked askew at Maggie. "Does that mean something to you?"

Maggie thought of the last time she'd seen Al. *A fisherman.* A flash of a memory came through. Was it six months ago? It hadn't been much more than that, certainly. Al and Maggie in their bathrobes on a waterfront balcony. Maggie's feet resting on Al's knees, Al's hands tracing circles along Maggie's ankles.

"Maybe, I, um. I don't know. So, what happened next? Has anyone spoken with her?"

Jess and Marcus were silent.

To be a doctor is to be a master of deductive reasoning, to be presented with a small set of disjointed facts and data that don't arrive in a linear or logical fashion, from an unreliable narrator. A doctor is a person who infers a cancer from a gaunt shadow under a cheekbone, a hand clutching a lower abdomen and a report of a night sweat. A person who knows certain things happen to certain people and unfold in certain patterns. A doctor should not need it to be spelled out. But Maggie did, in this moment.

"*Guys.* What. Happened."

Jess groaned and put her hands in front of her mouth, with the fingers separated just so to allow a thin sliver of air to pass through, as if this might filter the information of its poison quality.

"Well, then a few months ago Elizabeth got a message — Elizabeth runs the SocialEyes group you remember, the class president? — she got a message. From some relative of Alice. Brother, maybe? It said she had 'lost her battle with alcohol,' or something like that."

"*Lost her battle*? What does that really mean, though? What battle? What is a win or a loss?"

Marcus, losing patience with this exercise, leaned forward and looked Maggie directly in the eyes. "Maggie, she's dead. That's obvious, right? She's dead, is what that means. That's how you lose your battle with alcohol. That's the way."

Maggie was shaking her head, avoiding eye contact with her two colleagues.

"This simply isn't possible," she said confidently. "She sent me a text not that long ago." Maggie held her phone in her hand, but made no moves to challenge the statement with proof. "I just don't believe it," Maggie said. Her brow furrowed as her hand rubbed across it, her elbow resting on the table.

Al's hand resting on Maggie's calf, squeezing just a little. What if we move to Alaska, to work on a fishing boat? A little squeeze.

Maggie said quietly, to her own lap, "Does Al even *have* a brother?"

Jess and Marcus looked away in silence.

"I don't believe it," she said plainly.

Al, I took the job. Can we talk soon? That final message was still on Maggie's phone. Al had, eventually, responded with a thumbs up, Maggie was sure of it. It had taken a few weeks, but still. None of this made sense.

Marcus rolled his eyes, having had enough of these kid gloves. "Well, you can go ahead and not believe it, Mags, but no one has heard from her since, so just do the math, okay? The woman is dead."

A surgeon knows that a clean cut is best. A clean cut requires confidence and intention. A clean cut hurts just the same, but it heals better.

Maggie continued shaking her head. *I heard from her. Me, I did,* she thought but didn't say aloud.

Maggie's watch gave a buzz that brought her back to the present. *Orientation,* it reminded her. She flicked her wrist in annoyance, but the watch had a point. Breakfast was over. She was due elsewhere. There was work to do and thank god for that. She stopped shaking her head, neutralized her face, cleared her tears with a sleeve, and shuddered as if an emotional demon were being exorcized from her body.

"I gotta go. Orientation is starting. We should catch up more later, okay?"

Jess and Marcus nodded their assent, happy to be relieved of this burden for the time being. As Maggie rose from the table and turned to go, she felt the gaze of the nearby group of residents upon her and wondered how much of the conversation they had clocked. On the other hand, she probably didn't want to know. Just as she walked out of earshot, she heard the tail end of a conversation that perked her ears.

"Hey, you on anatomy lab duty tomorrow?"

"Ugh, yeah. You?"

"Yeah."

"Your turn to bring the Zofran."

Maggie walked faster to get out of earshot before she could hear more. As she left, she found herself reflexively scanning the room as she had on the way in, but she caught herself, shook her head, and moved on. Her head turned back one last time for good measure, and she shook it again.

The smell dissipated as Maggie walked out the door, but she could still taste it on her tongue.

Al is dead, she tried to comprehend, *but Al cannot be dead. Al is dead,* she repeated in her head, trying to overwrite the code in her brain that kept telling her otherwise. *Al is not dead,* as she pulled out her phone to check for the presence of that last texted *thumbs up. Al is definitely not dead,* as she touches the image with her own finger, as if it could become more real in the act. *Sent three months ago,* she noted. It had somehow seemed like less time than that; Al had never been a prompt text responder. It hadn't seemed like an unusual gap in communication. They had both been waiting, Maggie thought, for her arrival back in town. They were going to talk soon.

Al ain't dead. She left the lounge and shuffled down the hall, and her heavy Dansko'd feet kept the time of this repeated statement. *Al ain't dead.* Kerthunk kerthunk. *Al ain't dead.* Kerthunk kerthunk. *Al ain't dead.* Kerthunk kerthunk, like one of those meditative Buddhist mazes, her brain stuck in a loop of rumination that was rendering the words more meaningless with each repetition. *Al is Al is Al is Al is Al.*

The trance took her back to the beginning, where all this had started.

CHAPTER 2

MEDICAL SCHOOL YEAR ONE (MS1), FOURTEEN YEARS AGO.

On day one of medical school, the lungs of not-yet-doctor and not-yet-smoker Maggie Owens burned as she slogged up the steep grade to the hospital. *Why did they have to build this place on a hill,* she thought, resigning herself to the thought of four years of involuntary cardio that was probably good for her.

Why did they build this place on a hill? It was a question many had asked over the years. Students like her who were trudging uphill in the early hours, nauseated laboring women navigating the winding road to get there at two AM, frustrated parents looking for parking with a screaming and febrile child in the backseat. *Why?*

Truth was, the location had once seemed ideal back when illnesses were considered moral failings to be hidden away from the good people of a healthy society, a time when the primary cures for disease were fresh air, nature, and mercury. It was a time when the precarious horse-carriage ride up to the top of the hill was safer than the treatment rendered within the building. There might have been an opportunity forty or fifty years ago to start over in another more logical location, but instead they'd doubled down, taking over the hilltop with a patchwork of mismatched buildings and very little parking. Students weren't allowed to park on campus, one of the many ways in which Maggie would be reminded of her low-tier status over the next four years, and so Maggie had found a neighborhood behind the backside of the hill where she could stow her car and walk the remaining distance. The public bus system could have taken her to the front door, but having grown up in a place without such urbanity, she'd never ridden a public bus in her life and didn't imagine she'd want to start now.

Maggie tried to look at the bright side: maybe her sad calves would develop some definition for once in her life. Near the hospital's main entrance, Maggie stopped for a moment to admire an ornate fountain that bubbled up from the center of the large grassy courtyard that anchored the campus, taking up an unlikely amount of real estate for a place so otherwise cramped. *Great place for a parking garage if you ask me,* thought Maggie, as her calves continued to burn. She heard her mother's voice in her head, *Keep yourself fit, you never know when you'll meet your husband.*

This one's for you, mom, Maggie thought, grunting with each step.

She held a hospital map in one hand and her new white coat clutched in the other, inadvertently wrinkling the coat and dampening it with nervous palm sweat. She followed the general flow of people through the hospital entrance, glancing intermittently down at the map and its instructions. *Follow the signs for the green elevators and take them down to floor M.* Her shoulders sagged with the weight of her backpack's contents, $600 worth of textbooks whose heft was compressing (she would soon learn) the accessory nerves that ran beneath her trapezius muscles, causing an electric pain to radiate into her shoulders. Eventually she would also learn the real lesson at hand, that these books were largely unnecessary, especially not at the seven percent compounded student loan interest rate being placed on all her purchases at the moment. On day one, though, the burden of them felt grounding and real.

On the elevator, she stood at the back and re-adjusted her pack, now conscious of the space it occupied as the car filled with a mix of teetering elderly patients, tired residents and nurses, and a handful of other bright-eyed young people also clutching stark white coats and weighty backpacks. On the way down, the elevator car stopped and dropped and lurched and swayed, showing its age. Maggie clutched the strap of her backpack and took some deep breaths, wondering if this ride would get easier or harder over time. As they made their way down, passengers slowly trickled out until the only remainders were the fellow backpacked and white-coated, heading all to floor M, which seemed to be a mile below the earth's surface based on the darkness that fell over the car as it descended.

Several of the elevator's occupants seemed to know each other already, bantering in that blustery way that medical students do, dropping their resume into the conversation. *You guys will love Dr. Constantine. I was a research assistant in his undergrad lab. Small world, I was next door in the Johnson lab! Get out, my dad worked with Dr. Johnson before he became the department chair. My dad, that is.* The elevator shuddered as it passed into the sub-basement levels, and someone remarked *did you know this hill is supposedly a dormant volcano* right before it came to a halting stop. There was nervous laughter as doors opened, followed by the brief and awkward west-coast dance of everyone telling everyone else they should go first. Finally, when the doors threatened to close them all back in, the bolus of them spewed out all at once into the hallway. (Was bolus the correct term for a group of medical students? A phlegmon, perhaps? Or a grunt?)

The group made more small talk as they shuffled together down the long hall toward a set of double doors. *Don't you live in the Daniel?* one of them said to another, referring to one of the new condo buildings on the waterfront. *Yes, I think I saw you on the rooftop the other day.* Someone else said excitedly, *I'm in the Olivia across the street, maybe we could throw a zip line across* and there was more laughter. *Does everyone here live on the waterfront?* someone asked, and against her better judgment Maggie found herself saying *actually I'm renting a room on the other side of the river.* The condo-dwelling asker smiled kindly and said, *oh, that's cute,* as if Maggie's decision to rent a room far from campus were part of some boho chic aesthetic rather than an actual necessity of her poverty. The group came upon the double doors, which bore a red STOP sign and a badge reader next to them. The (*bezoar?*) of students all fell over themselves whipping out freshly-pressed badges to swipe at the reader, and the doors clicked loudly and split open, inviting the group into another long hallway that seemed to stretch out to an endless horizon.

Just beyond the entrance, two locker-room doors on either side of the hall split the group into two. On the left-hand side, the door showed a pants-wearing figure understood to be *MALE*. On the right-hand side was the hoop-skirted outline of a woman wearing clothing that would be fairly inconvenient attire for medical practice, and yet Maggie and the other students who understood themselves to be *FEMALE* headed into it anyhow.

Inside the door, Maggie found a women's locker room modest in size, with rows of worn lockers flanked by low benches, opposite a wall of unwelcome mirrors that promised to watch these women as they aged in fast forward over the next term. This locker room, they would later discover, was about half the size of the men's, in spite of the fact that well over half of the class had walked through its doors, a ratio that had held true for many years at this point. The door had that outline with the hoop skirt on it, though, so this is where these people go, no matter how many of them there are. This is the order of things.

Owing to its limited capacity, the room was already crowded. Scattered messenger bags and textbooks clustered on the floor, next to women in various states of undress. Though Maggie knew this was what locker rooms were like, she still felt jarred by it. She surveyed the room, trying not to cast her eyes too high or too low to meet the accidental gaze of a body part or an eye, and eventually saw that a table was set up on the far end with piles of blue-green scrubs. The other women in the room were changing while chatting, some standing absent-mindedly in bras and underwear asking casual questions like *where did you do undergrad* and *have you ever seen a dead body before* as if it were a perfectly normal situation.

Was this an unusual way to meet one's future colleagues? Of course. You would think they could have started with something less exposed, more dignified. A welcome breakfast. A luncheon. A tea party. A lecture hall, even. Those things were scheduled of course, more official and staid social activities for the new students. However, diving into the dissection lab day one had been a tradition of the school for decades now, and it served a purpose.

One day soon, they'll be inserting IVs into one another's veins for practice and crying to each other on the phone in the middle of the night because they can't memorize the Kreb's cycle; what does it matter if they know each other's preferred brand of panties. One day they will trade off chest compressions in the trauma bay, straddled atop a motorcycle crash victim, covered in blood, being yelled at by an ER attending to *push hard and push fast;* so what if they see some boob on day one. Someday, one will be diagnosed with breast cancer and will find another of these classmates standing over them at the operating table, ready to expose not just the outer but the inner confines of their diseased breast, and this will be a classmate who held their hair as they threw up behind a downtown bar after a bad breakup in year two, and who can sing all the words to *Informer* with complete fidelity, so they'll know they can trust them. Undressing together on day one was just the first step in the progression of intimacies that would pass between them over the years.

But. Of course at the time, at first, it seemed unusual. This was the system, though, the system that made a doctor, and the system was producing doctors, wasn't it? So, you could say the system was working perfectly.

Maggie scanned the room, looking for a corner she could slide into with as little notice as possible, still trying not to see the bodies of these women but noticing anyhow that an above-average set of them seemed to have sub-five-percent body fat, and that many of them seemed to be changing out of cycling gear that suggested a love of voluntarily physical activity to which she could not relate. *At least I'll be walking every day,* she thought, as she headed towards the scrub table at the end of the room and tucked in next to another woman who was sifting through the pile.

As Maggie arrived, the woman said to the room: "How do you tell the sizes? The tags are so faded I can't make them out." She was holding up a scrub top that seemed to be neither the size nor shape of a real human body, something like a perfect square.

The woman was compact, put together, with immaculate bone structure and a friendly but serious face, and dark hair pulled into a smooth bun that suggested dance in her extracurriculars. She looked over at Maggie, who smiled at her and shrugged, not knowing what to say. An answer came from behind them.

"God, those scrubs are so terrible, the size doesn't matter. If you want anything even remotely flattering you gotta buy your own and get them *tailored*." This statement came from a woman who was actively applying lipstick using a mirror inside one of the lockers. It seemed the woman had taken her own advice, based on the nipped waist of her own top.

Another woman behind Maggie scoffed, saying under her breath, "Nah, don't buy scrubs for Gross Anatomy, I hear they smell so bad by the end of the quarter they literally send them to the incinerator. Just get the largest ones and cinch the waist, no problem."

The lipstick woman, having heard this, added, "You know the anatomy preceptors are surgical residents right? I'm not showing up in those trash bags. You never know who you might need a rec letter from. You gotta look *profesh*."

The tailored-scrubs advocate had platinum blonde hair that fell with a heft and bounce that suggested pedigree; Maggie's own thin and shaggy ponytail was certainly not going to be having scrubs tailored. The forgiving spaciousness of scrubs was by design, she figured, what with the tendency of medical student life to expand and contract bodies depending on their call schedules and stress-eating habits. Maggie held a pair of pants up to her waist, considered whether her end-of-summer hips would fit comfortably within, and decided to give it a go. The much-smaller woman next to her grabbed the same size, giving Maggie a look as if to say, *us curvy girls gotta stick together*, which didn't seem an appropriate sentiment from what Maggie could see of this woman's narrow frame, but it made her feel understood, anyhow.

"Hi, I'm Maggie, by the way. Maggie Owens." Maggie had been

instructed by her mother that she should be more outwardly social now that she was going to be a doctor. She hoped this counted.

"Oh hey! Another O! I'm Jess Oliver! I think we're table mates, they assign them alphabetically."

Maggie smiled purposefully, repeating the name as she'd been told to do to help her remember. "Jess? Nice to meet you, Jess. Is that short for Jessica?"

"Ugh, JessieLynn actually. My family are country people." Jess was whispering close to Maggie's ear, as if they were already confidantes. "Don't tell anyone, no one will take a doctor seriously who has a country name. I'm hoping to legally change it before I graduate so it doesn't go on my medical license. Oh look, a couple of lockers are open over there, c'mon!"

Jess led the way, holding Maggie by the elbow softly. "Can you believe they make us do this shit on the first day? It's like junior high gym class, I had to buy new underwear just so I wouldn't be embarrassed. Let's just stay back in a corner and limit our exposure to mirrors."

Maggie had not purchased new underwear and had not even considered the implications of her underwear choice for that day. A quick panicked peek under her waistband reminded her of the flower-print boy shorts she had chosen. Not fashionable, but at least they would cover her ass, so to speak. She hoped Jess, who was already de-pantsed to expose high-cut Calvin Klein bikini bottoms, wouldn't judge.

Maggie hoisted her backpack into the locker, setting her hope-fully-too-big-and-not-too-small dissecting scrubs on the bench behind her. She slid her pants down with a deep breath, hoping that it wouldn't take long for this to feel less weird to her. Jess didn't seem fazed by it. Maggie imagined Jess must have played high school sports.

"Did I hear you say you're living on the east side? How did you get here?" Jess said, as she took off her top to reveal a matching Calvin Klein push-up bra. For a second, Maggie (disoriented by the sudden boobs, perhaps) interpreted the statement to be existential, like *how did a poor like you end up in a nice place like this*, before she realized what Jess was really asking.

"Like, what mode of transportation?" Maggie confirmed. Jess nodded, like *yeah, of course I mean what mode of transportation and not what life choices you dunce.*

"I drove. I had to park on the back side of the hill and walk up." Maggie tried to sound enthusiastic and positive as she added, "It'll be great cardio for me." She patted the roundness of her stomach as she said this in the way that women are taught to do when they talk about exercise, as if to acknowledge the exercise as penance for their excesses.

"Oh shit, we should carpool! I live up north, too. I got a sweet secret parking spot behind the convenience store two blocks away. I flirted with the manager there and he said I could use it. Who wants to live in those dumb condos, anyway? Boring rat cages if you ask me."

Maggie smiled in wonderment, nodding and saying *sounds great,* which indeed it did. She added, in a gossip whisper, "I'm just glad to find out I'm not the only one who can't afford to live on the waterfront, you know?"

"Girl, we don't have condos but we have survival skills, and that's way better."

"Yeah, yeah, way better."

Maggie was pretty sure she had neither a condo nor survival skills, and it wasn't clear why one would need to choose between the two, but she nodded anyhow, understanding that these kind of odd binaries do exist. Money versus Empathy. Legs versus Boobs. Smart Ones versus Pretty Ones.

Maggie's lot in that last binary had been cast by stringy medium-brown hair and an aggressively mid body that managed to be neither athletic nor curvy nor slender nor Rubenesque. *Who needs to be pretty when you're so smart,* the adults in her life would say as she grew up, especially after puberty, when they realized her cheeks were most likely just going to stay that round and her chest was likely going to stay that flat. Eventually they would start to pit her intellect against a potentially disastrous prettiness that really, truly, she had been lucky to have avoided. *Just be glad that you were born smart and not pretty* because smart is deep and forever and pretty is fleeting and shallow. *Good thing you aren't pretty, because then we would all have to hate you for having it too easy hahahaha.* Maybe you wouldn't have been pushed to score so high on the SAT, wouldn't have needed to read so many books, wouldn't have developed such a good sense of humor, because these are antithetical to being pretty. Just be glad you didn't end up outside the binary altogether, with the Leftovers. *I'm sure one day you'll find a husband that just loves your sense of humor,* her mother had said. *Maybe even a doctor,* she had added after Maggie was accepted to medical school.

Maggie tied up her scrubs and took stock of the fit. Not generous, but not uncomfortable. Jess, in the same size, was completely hidden by billowing fabric. The locker room was emptying out as people headed over to the dissection lab, and Maggie started to grab her backpack to join them. Jess stopped her.

"Girl, leave your books in the locker, you don't want to stink them up with *dead-body* smell. They've got laminated dissection guides for us there."

How was it that Jess seemed to know these ropes on day one? In fact, how was it that *everyone* seemed to have insider knowledge that she did not possess? Maggie was certain she had read every email (she had printed them out, in fact, three-hole punched them, and put them into a binder labeled *Medical School*). And yet, everyone else seemed to be in on some kind of insider secret, seemed to be wearing their scrubs so confidently and effortlessly while hers felt like a costume.

"Thanks Jess," said Maggie to her new (hopefully) friend. "I'm glad you're here to keep me straight."

Jess gestured for Maggie to follow her toward the door. "No problem, we gotta stick together, you know? It's going to get worse before it gets better, right?"

As they arrived in the dissection lab for the first time, the odor hit Maggie with more force than she'd been prepared for. Having grown up in midwestern farmland, the odor of organic decay was familiar; compost, manure, roadkill baking in the hot sun, skunk musk in the breeze. The lab odor had elements of those things, but was more twisted, angular. Somewhere in the uncanny valley between preservation and decay. Not the clean, chemical smell she had been anticipating. Unsettled. Aggressive.

Confusingly, it made her feel a little hungry. The hunger in turn brought nausea, and the hunger and the nausea fought each other for control of her stomach as she dug her fingernails into her palms and looked to the far wall. The room was, in theory, white on all sides, but with a faded quality, hinting toward a prior era when tobacco smoke might have filled the room. There were no windows, only fluorescent track lighting turned up just too bright for comfort, because comfort is not an affordable luxury when you need light enough to distinguish omentum from pancreas from thoracic duct from your own gloved hands. A low mechanical hum from the air handler softened all the hushed and anxious first-day chattering that otherwise would have echoed around its bare corners. Rows of metal tables held human forms concealed by long white sheets, some with toes just peeking out, like the first reveal in a macabre burlesque. Students were moving from table to table, examining clipboards at the foot of each table before eventually stopping at one. Some held their hands clasped in front of their chests like surgeons as they stood, observing an imaginary sterile operating field for which it was either too early or way too late. She suspected that a few people with downcast eyes may be praying, and others fighting back nausea as she was.

Jess was guiding Maggie toward a back corner by the elbow, a physical touch she normally wouldn't have appreciated, but that she was grateful for right now. They collected thick white notebooks labeled *GROSS ANATOMY: DISSECTION GUIDE* from a table near the entrance, the covers worn at the edges and stained in a way that suggested they had *seen things* and would *keep seeing things* for years to come. Maggie's misplaced hunger roiled in her stomach and her brow furled and her eyes watered.

"Here we are!" Jess said as they arrived at their table. She looked over and registered Maggie's pained expression. "Are you okay?"

Maggie shook her head. "The smell. . ." was all she could comfortably get out.

"No shit! Here, take some of this, it'll help." Jess palmed a tiny travel container of Vicks Vap-o-Rub into Maggie's hand. "Someone in the SocialEyes group recommended it." Jess saw Maggie's perplexed look, adding, "It goes under your nose, silly. Supposedly works wonders." Maggie did as she was told, and a wave of menthol overcame her, displacing the smell. The menthol also made her eyes water, but was a less nauseating burn.

Maggie passed the container back and asked, "What SocialEyes group?"

"You know, the class SocialEyes group?"

Maggie's face remained blank.

Jess gasped. "Oh my god, are you not in the SocialEyes group? You've *gotta* be in the SocialEyes group. We started it, like, *months* ago. I'll get you an invite, remind me later."

"Thanks," said Maggie. *How was I supposed to know about the SocialEyes group?* It was like one of those dreams where you arrive on test day having not been aware you were enrolled in the class. What other important information had she already missed?

"You know this smell? It's why all the first year students end up dating each other," Jess said, looking around the room. "Because *we* are going to smell like this soon. We'll have no other options but each other."

Maggie scrunched her nose up and shook her head vigorously.

"Ha, no thanks. To dating, I mean. I don't need *that* in my life, you know what I mean? I just ended something. I mean, it ended. It wasn't. . .I mean, you don't need to hear about that, sorry." Was oversharing also a side effect of formaldehyde inhalation, like hunger and nausea?

"Oh, honey! We are going to know ALL the secrets by the time this is over. I hear the formaldehyde is an aphrodisiac, too." Jess retightened the drawstring on her scrubs and threw her shoulders back slightly as she said this. Maggie was trying to parse Jess' face for signs this was a joke when a voice startled her from behind.

"Should I take an arm or a leg?"

Maggie jumped just a bit, and her hand knocked against the table, causing their cadaver to jiggle in a tiny shock wave and Maggie's own body to stiffen for a frightened split second.

"Oh, sorry! Didn't mean to scare you," the voice said, coming around the other side of the table to take its position next to Jess. "I guess you guys are stuck with me, sorry in advance. I'm Al."

"Alice, you mean?" Jess said. "Alice Power?"

The woman nodded, shrugged, then smiled. "I go by Al, but yeah."

"I recognized you from the SocialEyes group," said Jess. "Nice to meet you in person."

Alice Power.

Maggie would remember this moment, years later, the first time she saw Alice. Alice Power's name was one of those that evokes the form of what it is, like *The White House* or *The Hand of God;* a name where you lay eyes upon it and think, *yeah, that sounds about right.* Al's hair was thick, impossibly black, and stood up in pompadourian swirls and swoops above her head in defiance of gravity. She had a wide mouth that consumed her face when she smiled, and a sculpted, angular nose that seemed to point right at you when she spoke. Over-all, her face was just the most of everything, a maximalist study in human features. A face that was *captivating,* that stole your gaze, like one of those movie stars who shouldn't be handsome except for the fact that they are. Adam Driver. Benedict Cumberbatch. Tilda Swin-ton. Crispin Glover. People with an *it factor,* a way of bending the light in their direction from every angle, like a gravity well. You've seen these people in your life. You know when they walk into the room: they are *something.* Covered in whatever the human analog to Royal Jelly is.

Maggie felt herself become smaller, and smaller, and smaller in Al's presence. *If this is a person who is meant to be a doctor,* Maggie thought, *who the fuck am I?* Still, Maggie felt somehow lucky to be standing in her penumbra.

Al reached a hand across the shrouded form on the table to offer a handshake to Maggie. As she reached over, she patted the leg of the cadaver and said, politely, "Pardon my reach, sir," as if the body would or could take offense.

"What makes you so sure it's a sir?" Maggie asked, shaking Alice's hand in a way that she hoped was firm enough. "We don't know that yet."

"Oh, YES WE DO," Jess interjected. Her eyes gestured toward a swelling in the fabric midway down that gave it away. "And how!"

Indeed, it was a rather — impressive — profile. *Oh my,* Maggie mouthed and covered her eyes in faux-modesty. At this point, Alice produced a full-belly guffaw that seemed to Maggie to be a complete breach in decorum (*Was anyone else laughing,* she thought, *no one else seems to be laughing*), and Maggie held her finger up to her lips as she actively suppressed her own mirth.

The forces at play here were inciting a powerful conflict within Maggie's viscera that reignited her nausea. The awe-striking aura of Al's unstoppable visual confidence. The reinforced and immovable brick boundaries of Maggie's midwestern decorum. The nuclear humor of a dead man with a visibly over-sized penis on the table between them, the nauseating odor all around everything, the gaseous distention in Maggie's lower bowels that warned her she would need to release a fart at some point in the near future.

If I time it right, I can probably blame the smell on the dead guy, at least, she thought. That final thought broke her, and she gave up and joined in the laughter. If you can't laugh when you're meeting a group of strangers over a well-endowed dead guy's body, when can you laugh?

The laughter felt good, and she noticed that her hunger and nausea had been dissolved by it, even though *the smell* had actually grown stronger, as if their specific cadaver was in fact its epicenter. When the laughter died down, she noted, too, that her fart had dissipated into the mirth (she hadn't heard it or felt it go, but certainly it must have) and she sighed in relief while wiping an invisible tear away. Alice seemed to be looking at her — directly — in a way that people *like her* did not typically look at people *like Maggie.* Was she onto her about the fart? Did Maggie have something on her face? She subtly wiped the back of her hand under her nose to check for boogers.

Trying to find her way back into the polite society that the other groups seemed to be occupying, Maggie struck up some small talk, working off a list of questions her mom had suggested. *Where are you from? Do you have any hobbies or pets? What is your favorite TV show?* It still didn't come naturally to Maggie, but being the asker of questions (she had found) prevented her from needing to reveal too much of herself. (This feature was indeed part of the appeal of medicine as a career in general; the idea she could just disappear into the background of other people's stories.)

She didn't need to make it very far into the list, because first-year medical students love to talk about themselves. It is their primary skill thus far. On the first question alone, Maggie learned Al was from Texas, but she had gone to college *oh, near Boston, you know* for undergrad, and that she had already been published as the second author on a biomedical research paper entitled *Long-term Cold Storage, Pleiotropic Effects, and Drosophila Mating Behavior.*

"You haven't lived until you've spent four hours in the middle of the night thawing out fruit flies so they can fuck, amirite?" Al said proudly. "Anything for science, you know?"

"Is that what you guys were up to in your secret societies or whatever you call them over there?" Jess countered, adding that *as a Smith graduate*, she knew the Harvard faculty were prone to publishing junk papers just for pre-med undergrads to get their name on something.

"Wait," said Maggie, "Al, you went to Harvard?" She was sure she had been paying attention, and couldn't believe she'd have missed that detail.

"Of course she did, you doofus. That's what people mean when they say they went to college *'near Boston.'* She's trying to be coy about it."

"Oh," said Maggie, her body becoming impossibly small in midwestern state school ignorance. "That's funny."

Jess egged Alice on. "C'mon, Al. I know you're just *dying* to tell us about why frozen fruit flies fucking is somehow a relevant scientific breakthrough."

Alice took on a look of faux-offense, jaw dropped, eyebrows scowling, but somehow still smiling underneath. "*Cryogenics,* baby. You know there are hundreds of people in cold storage *right now,* waiting for science to catch up? Eventually, when we're curing all kinds of diseases with stem cells, we thaw them out, wake 'em up, *boom! Immortality."* Maggie found herself nodding, this making a kind of sense to her.

"Yeah!" Maggie said excitedly. "And then, *of course,* those unfrozen people are naturally going to be super horny."

"Exactly!" Al's blue eyes reflected the fluorescent overhead light right back into Maggie's eyes, momentarily blinding her. "Exactly. That's where the pleiotropic effects come in."

Maggie truthfully did not know what pleiotropic effects were, having never heard the word pleiotropic before, but nodded along anyhow. To ask what it meant, she feared, would show her hand as someone who *did not belong here,* which of course she did not, *of course,* having not gone to Harvard or Smith or any school with inside jokes about it. *Oh, you know, I went to school outside Des Moines,* she pictured herself saying to this crowd. *Oh shit, you went to Iowa State?* Al might say, before letting out a low, extended whistle. *God, you Iowa State girls, always trying to be so coy, just come out and say it.*

Listening to Alice and Jess talk (*God, you Harvard girls are insufferable,* Jess said), Maggie had growing concern that perhaps she had been admitted to the school to fulfill some kind of quota for nongeniuses that had been put into place to provide a buffer for the real medical students. *Twenty percent of medical students will drop out within the first year.* A friend in college had dropped that fact on her at one point, trying to talk her out of the harebrained idea of even applying. *It's all a money-making racket, is what it is.* At the time, that had sounded absurd to her, but now she was wondering. Was she here to be a kind of cannon fodder, destined to an early med-school grave?

"*I wonder where Christopher is —*" Jess was saying across the table, pointing at the last name on the clipboard who was not yet present.

Al shrugged. "Probably chickened out when he saw the student loan paperwork. There's a couple every year." Al laughed again, and so Maggie laughed again, and everyone was laughing, except Maggie wasn't really laughing, because she herself had nearly ended up in this statistic a month ago, when she had sat and stared at the five-figure sum on her own student loan paperwork in disbelief for three days before closing her eyes and just signing it. Coming from the open plains of a midwestern small town, the loan amount had felt impossibly high — more than her parents' entire house was worth — and with no guarantee that she'd even make it past the first semester.

Twenty percent of medical students drop out in the first year, she had thought, before holding her breath and signing. *But it can't be me.*

The signature had put a final end to the barrage of calls in the preceding month from military recruiters offering to put her through school for free in exchange for conscription. The calls came in the evenings from handsome-sounding men who would whisper sweet nothings in her ear as she cooked ramen noodles in her hot-plate studio kitchen. *See the world,* they had said. *No malpractice,* they had said. *You'll be debt free and building wealth when your classmates are a half million in the red.* She would respond, *but I don't want to fight, I want to heal,* meekly, with an unwitting giggle, *that's why I want to be a doctor.* They would counter, *The Navy is about peacekeeping! The United States Army is the most diverse workforce in the nation! Women are an integral part of leadership in the modern Marines!* Maggie had heard them out, these fit and muscular and desperate men, because a midwestern woman is polite and accommodating, and because she liked the imagined world they were selling to her as much as she knew it to be a fraud, and because when else in her life would she have so many men so interested in talking to her for so long. She had continued to take the calls far longer than her actual interest in military enrollment had extended, but eventually she had to fess up that she just couldn't do it. *Your loss,* one annoyed recruiter had said when she told him to stop calling, *good luck with all your loans and your boring life. Thanks,* she had said in return, *thank you so much.* A midwestern woman can take neither a compliment nor an insult.

The room was quieting as a distinguished-looking man (read: bald, white, older, wearing a white coat) stood upon a step stool at the front of the room, raising two hands in the air as an orchestra conductor might. His well-rested and confident gaze provided a foil for the phalanx of people who flanked him on either side, wan bodies who somehow looked both younger and older than the man, forms who had the appearance of people whose physical bodies had remained behind after their souls had escaped, like whatever the opposite of a ghost is. Their hair was disorganized, dull, thin, limp. Their orbital bones seemed to be visible, somehow, and beneath them were hollowed and darkened spaces that seemed to suck the light out from their bloodshot eyes. *Those must be the surgical residents*, Maggie thought, recognizing this aesthetic as one that is often worn with pride in a teaching hospital, as it marks the accomplishment of having successfully banished sleep and self-care from one's life, of having thoroughly transformed one's body into a vessel for the practice of medicine and nothing else.

"*I think those are the surgical residents,*" Alice was whispering to the table, gesturing in that direction. "*Look sharp!*" She stood up a little taller, with exaggerated posture.

"*Yeah, look sharp, Maggie! Don't forget your tailored scrubs!*" Jess added, comically cinching the waist on her scrub pants and sticking her chest out for effect. Maggie laughed at the thought that these sad people might somehow notice a fitted pant. Then again, what did she know? Maybe that was the only thing they had the energy to notice these days.

The bald man at the front was talking now. No doubt, a speech to first-year students on the first minute of the first day that he had honed over years upon years upon years. Just enough gravitas and pomp and circumstance, mixed with a smattering of practicality. *Congratulations on being here,* he said. *This is the first day of an experience that will change who you are.* He referred to the profession of medicine as a *centuries-old fraternity,* reminded them they had been selected *from an accomplished pool of over five thousand applicants, all of whom would love to be in your spot right now* and they represented the best and the brightest minds in the country. Maggie shrank a little as he said this, wondering if he was leaving out an unspoken qualifier, *except for those of you who we only admitted so you could pay us 60 thousand dollars to flunk out.* He also told them to show up dressed appropriately, with long hair tied back and nails trimmed short. *You are adults now. You need to show up on time and ready, of your own accord. No one here is going to hold your hand.*

Just as he made the last statement, the double doors at the front of the room opened gingerly, and a tall and curly-haired head poked through the opening with a sheepish look. Dr. Bald Man cleared his throat and gestured over to the latecomer. "I see we have a case in point! So nice of you to help me demonstrate it for the class. Come on in, sir. Your table will be the one with only three people at it."

Jess raised her hand to call the figure over to them. "Back here!"

The rest of the class tittered.

The man presumed to be Christopher strode over to them with the muted confidence of a person who was used to being visibly late to things, and took his spot next to Maggie. He had a face that was round and soft, and a body to match. Tall, probably strong, but not too angular or defined, not overly attractive but fine enough to look at. His skin seemed a bit more weathered than was appropriate for his age, like perhaps he'd grown up on a farm, or had spent the summer hiking the Pacific Crest Trail or something. Maggie gave him a tiny wave hello as he came to stand next to her.

"*Sorry I'm late,*" he whispered as Dr. Bald Man was continuing on. "*My truck wouldn't start this morning and I had to walk.*" The imagery of him sitting in the cab of a weathered old Ford Ranger with a dead battery completed Maggie's assumptions about a farm-land upbringing.

I'll bet he's not even part of the SocialEyes group, Maggie thought, happy to have someone else be even more of an outsider. Her mom's voice cut into her smug satisfaction, saying *you never know when you'll meet your husband.* Maggie gave Christopher a smile that she hoped was perceived as welcoming.

The bald man wrapped up with some specific points about the treatment of cadavers. *Treat them with respect, like they're your own family members,* he said, as if the methodical removal of body parts was a type of thing you might visit (respectfully) upon one's own family member. *Don't mind me, Mom, I just need to take a look at your flexor pollicus longus. I won't be much of a bother. Do you think we can get sushi after?* Or, *many apologies, Uncle Joe, but I will have to uncover your cremaster muscle this afternoon, awkward but I promise we can turn on the game when we're done.* Not happy to leave anything the least bit unclear, Dr. Bald Man went on to provide specifics. *Do not desecrate the cadavers. Do not carve your initials into them. Do not use them for practical jokes. Do not insult their bodies excessively.* Maggie wondered about the qualifier of *excessively*, like *some is inevitable but don't get carried away.*

There was surely precedent for Dr. Bald Man to have to say these things to these buttoned-up medical students who had suppressed all joyful impulses for years to get to this point. Certainly he'd seen the pressure boil over enough times over the years. He didn't explicitly bar laughter or mirth, but Maggie still gave Alice a look like *are you listening to this* from across the table, and Al gave her a smiling little salute in response.

Dr. Bald Man got right into more practical considerations. How to assemble the scalpel blades, how to hold them (*like a pencil, we aren't chopping vegetables here*), basic dissection safety etiquette, how to keep the body moistened with preservative-soaked towels as they worked, how to divide up tasks among themselves. *Luckily, most of the parts are duplicated, so it's easy to share.* Proof of divine design or evolution, depending on your perspective.

Then, the moment they had been waiting for. The group donned gloves from racks under the tables, Al pulling hers down and snapping them for effect as she looked Maggie in the eye. Maggie made a point this time not to laugh, deciding not to further encourage this kind of tomfoolery. They were instructed to bring the sheets down to half-mast, *just down to the waist, NO LOWER,* as if preserving modesty were the utmost concern at a time like this. Jess and Maggie were given the honors of pulling the sheet down, owing to their position across the table near the head.

"Ladies first, we'll let you do the honors," Al said, winking at Maggie. Christopher had his hands clasped in front of him in reverence, mirroring the repose of their patient, whose hands were tied at belly-level with twine; Al's hands were spinning a scalpel handle between her fingers like a drummer during a set break.

Their first look at the body was jarring, somehow unexpected, even after the long anticipation that had led up to it. This had the shape of a human, the features of a living being, but was an *object* rather than a *subject.* Some stigmata of human life remained. Weathered skin, a sword tattooed across the chest, an arcuate scar upon one shoulder suggesting a prior surgery. A concave abdomen told a story about the man's last days, either starving or not hungry at all. The face remained shrouded, though Maggie already began to dread the day when it would be revealed.

The tattoo had already gotten to her, being so specific and personal, something that could be tied to a story and a feeling and a choice that this person, this *actual man,* had made in his actual life. Maggie's mind involuntarily began filling out a face to match the body. Unshaven, she guessed, with sunken cheeks to match the abdomen. Perhaps a scar across one eyebrow from a fishing accident or a bar fight. Teeth in disarray. Nose hairs grown out of turn.

This reverie was interrupted by the next task at hand. Since the dissection was to begin on the upper back, the group was forced to work together to turn the body over.

"Alrighty, let's get this show on the road," Al said, cracking her knuckles theatrically.

Christopher put a hand out to request a pause. He sucked in a long breath and let it out slowly. "How amazing is it that this man gave his body to us? Perhaps we could take a moment to give thanks."

Alice's face tensed into the not-smile formation that a person makes when a smile won't be welcome. Eyebrows and lids pulled upwards, with the mouth pulled straight back. Jess's face was similarly arranged, and Maggie had to make a point to avoid their gaze. She looked up at Christopher's earnest face, with kind brown eyes that looked as if they might produce a tear at any moment. A midwestern woman cannot deny a face like this, it isn't possible. In fact, they can't even try.

"You're right, Christopher," Maggie said, placing her one gloved hand upon the man's shoulder. "Thanks, guy." She found herself shuddering with the touch involuntarily. "Thanks a lot." Christopher nodded approvingly, then looked over at the other two across the table.

Alice nodded along in seeming solemnity, but a pointed eye contact and a telltale contraction in her brow sent a different message to Maggie. Al's eyes drifted south, to the cadaver's *ahem* prominent midline apex, and then back up.

"Thank you, sir. *Big* thank you," Alice said with a just-perceptible raise of one brow. Jess caught on to this and joined in.

"Oh yes, thank you for your service, *indeed*."

Jess, Maggie, and Alice all had faces screwed into suppressed laughter, Maggie feeling an actual pain at the conflict between her humor and her politesse, while Christopher, having missed the subtext of their comments and the earlier dick-size discussion, seemed blissfully unaware of the joke.

"Well, should we get to it?" he said, rubbing his hands together.

With that, the group took up their positions, wrapping their arms around the body in preparation for the flip.

"How did you guys know I'm an ass man," Al said as she managed the rump, while Christopher managed the legs and Jess and Maggie worked together on the shoulders.

"Ready," said Christopher, and they all nodded. He counted off, and on *three*, they all grunted with the effort.

It didn't go smoothly. The body was less rigid than expected, with toneless muscles and loosened joints that flew in the face of anyone who would refer to a dead body as *stiff*. As a result, instead of turning over in an orderly log roll, the body flexed at the waist and buckled into itself with their effort, briefly resting in something of a downward dog before crashing awkwardly onto the table while Christopher and Alice hugged the bottom half to keep it from ending up on the floor. During the maneuver, Maggie caught a glimpse under the sheet (Accidentally? *Mostly* accidentally? *Maybe a little* on purpose?), confirming the group's suspicions about the gentleman's endowment. She found herself not-totally-silently mouthing, *oh wow*, before she could stop it. Alice, whose eyes had been on Maggie even as she wrangled the flailing rump, caught her looking. Maggie blushed, then shrugged, stifling the impulse to make a silly comment. The act of stifling the comment gave her a pained look, like one holding in a sneeze. Alice noticed the look and gave a knowing one in return.

These looks quickly turned sour when the smell hit. With the crash, a wave of *smell* had wafted up from under the sheet, having been released from the dutch oven in which it had apparently been trapped, adding to the pain.

"Well, THAT went well," Jess said, before screwing up her face with Alice and Maggie. "Good god, did someone fart?"

"Sorry," Maggie said, smiling. "It was me. I couldn't hold it any longer." That broke them, and the group started to giggle as quietly as they could muster, the cumulative effect of the smell and their anxiety and the crashing body too much to continue holding in.

Christopher looked back and forth between the rest of his group with concern. "Hey, I just want to remind everyone," he said with the authority that was afforded to him as a tall person, and the only man in the group, "that this human being is made from the same material as stardust." He was re-positioning the modesty drape over the body's lower half, straightening the sheet and smoothing out the wrinkles like a hotel housekeeper might.

"Sorry." Maggie blushed. "It's just nerves, you know. I can assure you we are taking this very seriously."

"Very seriously," echoed Alice, less convincingly.

With the body appropriately pronated, Maggie felt a sense of relief. The contours of the face and the chest and the tattoo and the *you-know-what* were now hidden on the underside, and the body had transformed into something more scientific and impersonal in their absence. They all stood for a second, looking at one another, at the body, at the dissection guide, at the tray of scalpels, at the other tables of students, back at each other. Maggie's hands hovered over the surface of the body without touching it, as if she were a gymnast about to start her beam routine. She couldn't bring herself to use the body to rest her hands, but also didn't know what else to do with them. Alice, as a counterpoint, was gripping an ass cheek through the sheet and leaning comfortably.

"All right people. Anyone else been practicing scalpel skills on chicken breasts all summer, or should I make the first cut?" Al gave the glute a little goose with her hand as she said this.

Maggie had spent her summer working double shifts as a server at a 24-hour diner in Omaha, having been unaware that she might have used the time for something else. *Day one, and I'm already behind, just great.* She looked across the table at Jess to see if she was feeling similarly out of depth. Jess whispered back at her across the table.

"Don't worry about it, Maggie. We've just got a gunner on our hands."

Alice puffed up her chest at the term *gunner*. "If I'm going to be Dr. Power, I can't help it, you know?"

Gunner was another term that Maggie had not heard before, at least not used outside a wartime context. *Gunner* was an inside word that had been redefined at some point in the past, probably by a single med student, who had then posted it on some online forum like *studentdoctor.net*, where it spread to the far corners of med student parlance everywhere. *Gunner* referred broadly to a subset of medical students who were *out for blood*, who would eat their own and then brag about it, who would sell their own mother if it bumped their class rank up into the top quartile. A gunner buys coffee for some professors and flirts with others. A gunner keeps a full accounting of not just their own test scores, but of yours, too. A gunner is privy to the following Big Secret: that the amount of knowledge in this world is finite, and to increase your own cache, you'll need to wrest it from someone else's cold, desperate hands, and hide it away like a chipmunk in winter. Not so much Mr. Steal-Your-Girl as Mr. Steal-Your-Notes. *Gunner* was a term that implied success, but it was not at all a compliment. However, a gunner will take it as one. Al seemed to take it as such.

"I like to think of myself as more of a pilot, but if gunner gets me into the Surgery program at Mass General, I'll take it."

Jess rolled her eyes. "Harvard girls are so insufferable, right?" She looked at Maggie for agreement.

"Yeah," Maggie said, having no prior experience with Harvard people of any kind, "The worst." Al smiled at Maggie as she said this and wiggled her eyebrows up and down, since *being the worst* was a mark of honor to Harvard grads and gunners alike. Al was assembling her scalpel blade and examining her dissection guide, as Maggie and Jess gingerly palpated the spinous processes that were the landmarks for the first incision. Christopher was gazing down at the cadaver, his hands resting gently on the man's arm.

"We should name him." Christopher looked at Maggie when he said this, then at the other two.

"Yes, names are important," said Maggie.

Alice looked up from her scalpel assembly. "How about Chuck Norris?"

Jess shook her head. "No way, I don't want our cadaver rising from the dead to kick our ass, huh-uh."

"It's gotta be a name like that, though. A badass. A rebel. A loner." Al was right. The torso had told them enough about the type of man they were dealing with.

"How about Tommy," offered Jess. "After Tommy Lee." This drew a laugh from Al and a secret smile from Maggie.

"I don't think we can name him after a *living* person," said Christopher, missing the joke. "Bad karma."

The group quieted for a moment as they stared at the man's backside collectively, waiting for a name to reveal itself from its curves.

Maggie was the next to speak up. "How about just a regular name, like. . .I don't know, Frank?"

"Frank sounds good to me," affirmed Christopher. "Good, solid name." The group silently rolled the name *Frank* around in their minds as they took in the form with rough, tanned skin and well-developed deltoids. *Frank.* Frank is man who has lived a working life. *Frank.* Frank wears blue jeans and cowboy boots and a suit jacket without a tie. *Frank.* Frank works with tools and machines and might call you *sugar* or *little lady* but he doesn't mean anything bad by it.

"I'm good with Frank," Jess agreed.

Alice nodded along. Her eyes twinkled, and she held her scalpel up as if it were a gun. "What about, *Frank T. Blood, Private Eye.*" Christopher made a motion as if to object until Maggie interrupted him.

"Perfect," said Maggie. "Frank T. Blood, Private Eye. It's *perfect.*"

Al took the opportunity to ready the scalpel at the nape of Frank's neck. "Alright mister, no more secrets."

With that, she made the first cut, from C7 to T10, with one bold move that went straight down through the flesh to the spinous processes, just as the dissection guide had directed.

"That's how it's done, people," Al said. She gave Maggie a little wink, just Maggie and no one else, the first time a *Harvard girl* had ever winked at Maggie, and to Maggie it felt like this wink had admitted her to medical school as much as the admissions committee had.

The cut itself was not remarkable, being a straight line, but it was beautiful nonetheless — the flesh splitting open just enough to reveal the red sinew beneath (surprisingly red, in hindsight, *a little too red, even*), sparkling in the fluorescent glow of the overhead track lighting, the slightest bit of bright white bone peeking through at the base.

The proud satisfaction lasted just a moment, after which the faces of the four fell out of awe and into something more pained. Eyebrows pulled toward the center, lips pursing, noses turned just slightly to the side, as if that would somehow make a difference.

Jess was the first to speak up.

"Good GOD, what IS that *smell?*"

CHAPTER 3

PGY10

Al *is dead,* Maggie was repeating in her mind as she was whisked up to the eighth floor. *Al is dead.* She was still cycling through this mantra when the elevator doors opened and, with the impeccable comedic timing of the universe, Maggie was greeted by none other than Al herself.

Al's face, that is. It graced the center of a large photo mural that faced the elevator doors as Maggie entered the Department of Caregiver Training and Resources (abbreviated everywhere as DoCTR), where she was to be oriented that morning. The photo tableau featured a number of scrubbed and stethoscoped healthcare workers wearing broad, fanatic smiles that suggested a possible hostage situation at the photo shoot. Marcus' face was here too, predictably, part of a multiracial rainbow of faces that mostly were looking up and to the right, as if they were tracking a bird or a plane in the distance. *Looking for an exit,* Maggie thought. Al's face, though, was dead on. It's over-large mural-eyes bore down on Maggie as she stood there, slack-jawed. Maggie put her sleeve back up to her nose to filter the scent of foul air.

I'm dead, Al's face seemed to be saying to Maggie, as she turned away from it and started down the hallway. *I'm dead,* it seemed to yell at Maggie as she increased the pace of her steps. *I'm dead, so don't be late for orientation.*

You aren't dead, Maggie said back silently, trying to push the face and the contradicting voice out of her head. As Maggie walked, a dead-but-not-dead zombie Al rose out of her imagination, peeling right off the mural wall to follow her. Zombie Al was straight-arm-walking down the hallway, giving chase too slowly to catch up, saying *yooouuuu'll paaaaay foooor thiiiiiiis* in her best zombie voice.

Maggie shook her head to rid herself of the vision. Al wasn't a zombie, of course. Al was just dead, right? Along with billions of other humans dating back to whatever first hominid had forked off from the Neanderthals to walk fully upright. This was the way the system was set up, in a binary. Either. Or. But not both. Maggie was alive, and Al was dead. Maggie was alive, and she walked toward the DoCTR Conference Room with this truth rattling around in her brain. Al is dead. *Al ain't dead,* she thought again, as she rounded the corner toward her destination.

That morning, the trappings of a New Employee Orientation seemed utterly ridiculous. She could picture the scene before she even arrived: A sign-in table staffed by an overly cheerful woman wearing outdated makeup, a pre-printed name tag promising unwanted social interaction, a schedule full of ice-breaker activities like hospital scavenger hunts and hobby bingo and demands to tell the group two truths and a lie about yourself. A photo taken under unflattering lighting, a badge destined to open almost all the doors in the hospital except for the one supply closet you actually need access to. A badge with a photo that will fade and fade and fade with repeated use into a ghostly version of its owner, mirroring the aging of one's spirit, like a modern-day Dorian Gray. A stack of orientation papers that you feel obligated to take home in spite of knowing it to be garbage. Benefits breakdown. Hospital map. Employee Assistance Program brochure. The trees exist, so why not make the paper? The paper exists, so why not hold it for a while?

What if the two truths are that you've been drinking every night to stop your nightmares, and that you haven't seen a dentist in five years?

What if the lie is that you went into medicine to help people? Maggie thought these things as she pushed through the doors to the DoCTR.

A chipper woman in a pink suit behind the desk said good morning, and Maggie smiled silently back at her in a way she hoped would imply both politeness and a desire for no further conversation. Maggie, identified on the sign-in sheet as a physician, was handed a glossy packet for the Physician Wellness Program, and she laughed; in that way people laugh when something isn't funny. She stood for a second perusing the offerings: A series of classes called *Resilience Training*, described as *high-level burnout prevention strategies that work!* An online webinar series with the title *Attitude is a Choice*. An instruction sheet for something called *Progressive Relaxation in Motion!* An invitation to a *Lunchtime Yoga Series with Hazel*.

The backside of the packet was just a black-and-white sign that said YOU MATTER, and Maggie laughed again, as the woman in the pink suit pretended not to notice.

Perhaps Alice was given one of these packets, suggesting she do Yoga to recover from the collapse of her entire life. Maggie was overcome with rage at the idea, a rage she demonstrated by folding the packet in half, creasing the edges firmly with a nail, and tucking it neatly into her messenger bag.

Wellness Program, my ass. Was that a thought Maggie had or a voice she'd heard? *We can all be well when we're dead.*

A well physician (somewhere in a conference room an executive is making this joke) is just the opposite of a top shelf physician, amirite? A Wellness Program is never having to say you're sorry. Was there a smell growing in this room? Surely not. Maggie coughed and cleared her throat, pulling a mask out of her bag and onto her face.

She took her seat, putting both her phone and her ponytail in front of her masked face to try to look uninterruptible.

Buck, 48, High School Chemistry Teacher. Detention can be fun, I promise. Picture of him in handcuffs, wearing a ball gag. Swipe right. *Just what I need, I think.*

Someone next to her cleared their throat, and Maggie quickly turned the phone face down in her lap.

"You hear about all the fires?"

Maggie reflexively turned to her left with immediate regret. Her face met that of a smiling young person, early twenties at best, dressed in a dark polo shirt and pressed khakis, a shock of unruly blue hair atop their head, the look of a lead singer for a nineties ska revival band but make them a Best Buy employee. *Hello My Name Is Jax, They/Them* said their name tag. They had sat directly next to Maggie, in spite of the dozen other empty seats they could have chosen around the room.

Damn. A generation raised on Zoom calls, uneducated on the unwritten seating-rules of in-person meetings. A generation over-hungry for close-range eye contact.

"Pardon?" Maggie raised an eyebrow. She clutched the phone to her chest with one hand, as if to signal her intent to return to it at any moment.

"All those fires," said Jax. "The guy who's burning trash all over the city." Jax was pulling their mask down to talk, and Maggie subtly pinched the nose piece on her own.

"Oh, I wasn't sure if you were talking about that or the Amazon or what. Lotta fires to choose from these days."

"Amazon? The forest, you mean? Is that still a thing?" Jax's green eyes were darting not-subtly down to Maggie's chest and back again. Maggie gave them the benefit of the doubt as she realized the corner of her own name tag was hidden by her cardigan in just that location.

"Maggie," she said, pulling back the corner of her cardigan to reveal the tag underneath. "My name is Maggie." She paused, and added awkwardly, "Uh, She/Her." She not-so-subtly glanced at her watch (4 minutes until the thing started), then back at her phone.

"Hi Maggie, I'm Jax. I'm going to be doing IT support." Jax waited for Maggie to reciprocate, but she just stared, nodding, eyebrows up.

"That's cool. Good for you. That. . .makes sense." This might have been an insult, but Jax took it as encouragement.

"It's cool they're doing this thing in person, right? This is like, my only chance to even see the hospital. We all work remote now."

"Oh," said Maggie. She wasn't making eye contact, but she had a face that always seemed like it was listening, so it didn't matter.

Jax continued, "I was in a research lab before. *Drosophila*. Do you know what that is? It's fruit flies." This accelerating over-sharing did not bode well for the next 4 hours. Maggie found herself perversely looking forward to the cold silence of the afternoon, which was promised to online modules in the computer lab.

"Fruit flies need IT support?"

Jax laughed a little too generously at this, clarifying that the scientists needed the IT support, "not the flies, silly!" For statistical modeling and genome mapping. The fruit flies just needed sugar water, they thought.

"Or fruit, right?" Maggie offered. She shouldn't have continued making jokes, but it couldn't be helped. Jax laughed heartily again, wiping a few imaginary tears from their lower lids.

"Oh man, you're funny!" Jax was now slapping the table. *This generation really needs more human contact,* Maggie thought.

Jax continued, "Hey, so are you like a nurse or something?"

Maggie had a script that she had practiced for this situation, one that went: *No I'm Not a Nurse, though Nursing is a Fine and Noble Profession I am Something Else but Nurses Are Literally. The. Best.* Usually this was followed by a shrinking and shrugging apology, *Well, Actually I'm a Doctor, Not That Doctors Are Better Than Nurses But They Are Different.* In her head, she would add silently, *And They Can Sometimes Have a Vagina.*

Maggie found herself too tired to give it all this juice today and said instead:

"No, I'm not a nurse."

"Oh, shit, I'm sorry. I shouldn't have assumed. What are you, then?"

Maggie Owens, MD, said her name tag. Maggie glanced at it for a second, and then back at Jax, who didn't catch the hint. *Actually, I'm an introvert,* Maggie considered saying, but didn't. She just stared blankly, trying to delay the inevitable. Telling people you are a doctor, Maggie had found, was like telling someone you are a vegan, or that you went to Harvard, or that you have cancer. A bucket of ice water on any conversation.

Maggie was saved from answering as the pink suit arrived at the front of the room and clapped her hands together excitedly.

"Good Mooooooorning Everybody!!"

Maggie shrugged, smiled, and turned away from Jax, covering her name tag back up and putting her phone into her lap politely. The room's chatter faded to zero as the other introverts sighed a collective relief and turned their attention to the extrovert standing at the front. The woman had a tight brown haircut with well-placed highlights (you know the haircut, you know you do) and was dressed in a salmon-pink skirt suit, accessorized with a waxy, frozen smile. She seemed to make eye contact with everyone in the room all at once.

"*I said, GOOD MOOOOOOORNING EVERY-BOOOOODY!!!*"

The woman introduced herself as Debbie (*but you can call me DoCTR Debbie, she said*), and though Maggie had never met her, this was a person she knew well, that everyone in medicine knows well. PTA President, member of the HOA board, the type of person who, given a microphone and license, would yell at complete strangers to say Good Morning louder and louder until they pleased her. This person, with her aggressive smile, and her low heels, and her expensive haircut; this person was a Suit. She was part of a long line of Suits who sprung from other Suits who were molded in the Furnace of Suits that marked the Original Sin of the medical community. The Suits had not always been there. But the Suits were eternal, all the same.

In the beginning, there were the Coats, and the Coats were beloved. The Coats were all men, of course, and especially white men, and extra especially tall white men of an age with tailored beards they could stroke while talking to the Gowns. At first, the Coats did not have much to offer the Gowns, other than fresh air and black bags that clasped with a satisfying *clunk* and deep voices that could reassure them as they died of either consumption or the attempts to treat consumption. The Coats had those things, and they had gravitas, and that was enough for a world where the life expectancy was forty-five and most people died of *Oregon Trail*-inspired diseases like dysentery. Eventually, the coats also had scalpels, and then opium and ether to allow them to use the scalpels, and these were good things. And then came Penicillin, a Real Drug that Actually Worked and they added this to the fresh air and the black bags and the deep voices and the scalpels, and the ether, and the opium, (and a few other things that also turned out to basically be opium under further scrutiny), and the Coats finally had something to offer to the world. The Coats were kind of like scientists and kind of like priests, neither of which were particularly good at managing money or organizing schedules or making systems for distributing cure-alls like aspirin and penicillin and opium and more opium.

So they hired Suits to do those parts. The Suits didn't need to know anything about Aspirin or Penicillin or opium or drugs that were also opium or still other drugs that were extremely similar to opium. They just needed to know about money. And *boy did they know about money*. And the Suits worked for the Coats, at first. The Suits engineered more efficient ways to convince the Gowns to part with their money, and to feel good about it to report on surveys. And the Coats were getting the money, and the money was good. And the Money bought the Coats nice cars and big houses and so they didn't ask too much about it. Because the Coats were like scientists and like priests and it was taboo for scientists and priests to think about money, but that didn't mean it hadn't felt good to have it. And the Gowns started to love the Coats a little less, because they saw the nice cars and the big houses, (and a little bit because of all the things they were told were definitely-not-opium, but turned out to be exactly-one-hundred-percent-opium). But the Gowns still loved them enough, and everyone was happy.

Except the Suits. The Suits also saw the nice cars and the big houses and the Coats who were like scientists and priests who were not supposed to think about money. So the Suits hired more Suits, who hired more Suits, and they all got together to buy all the buildings and all the aspirin and all the black bags and all the scalpels and all the ether, until the Coats had to work for the Suits, because the Suits now owned the means of production.

And now? Now, the Suits stand up in front of crowds of Coats and tell them about the dress code and Medicare fraud and anti-kick-back-statutes and productivity expectations and they smile and they smile and they smile and they smile.

In the face of a Suit, Coats will often disappear inside themselves as a survival instinct. As such, Maggie caught only chops and screws of the next hour of content, having reflexively re-embarked on her *p*Value* expedition, holding her phone furtively in her lap and casting glances down at it when the pink suit had her back turned.

Chaz, 37, Cryptozoologist. Picture in complete shadow. *Sometimes the mystery is the best part.* Maggie swiped right, because why not?

DoCTR Debbie was giving an impassioned entreaty that no job was too small to contribute to the mission. *There are no hierarchies here. If you see something, say something. You know at Toyota, any employee can stop the line. Really! There are no hierarchies here! A doctor and a mailroom attendant are all contributing to the mission equally!* Was she looking at Maggie when she said this?

Smith, 44, Botany Entrepreneur. Grateful Dead t-shirt, cargo shorts, blonde mullet. Kind dimples. Definitely in the weed industry. Fuck it, swipe right. She'd already passed her onboarding drug test.

DoCTR Debbie relayed a story about a cafeteria employee whose scratch-made soups were so comforting to older patients, they'd added them to delirium prevention protocols, because *there are no hierarchies here, there really aren't.*

Jack, 34, Physician. Libra. Head shot wearing a white coat, stethoscope draped around his neck, mottled gray photo background she recognized from her own headshot taken last week. *For a good time, find me on KnockKnock! @dancindoctorjack! New video every week.* Another right swipe. Maggie had a storied history of shitting where she ate. Why stop now?

The suit was wrapping up. Sincere, intense. *You're part of this family now! If you don't wake up happy to come to work every day, I will take it as a personal affront! And you don't need a fancy degree to know that laughter is the best medicine, and a smile can save a life! Am I right? I said, AM I RIGHT?!* Applause from the room.

The simple optimism of an upper-middle-class white woman, unshakeable.

The rest of the morning passed quickly for Maggie, in a haze of *p*Value* shuffling, doom scrolling, daydreaming, and the occasional and brief forced interaction with Jax, who never caught on to Maggie's secret identity. A few minutes before the final speaker wrapped, a young man in a branded polo shirt pushed through the door into the room carrying a couple of bags that he began to unpack onto a side table. He was placing small boxes labeled *Giraffe and Co. Sandwich Company* into two sections on the table, and Maggie knew from experience that the lunch options in these boxes would be either an unusually outfitted turkey sandwich with cranberry sauce or a vegetarian hummus, cucumber, and mozzarella on focaccia, both with a piece of sad fruit and a tiny bottle of water that was stopping here on its way to a giant garbage patch in the middle of the Pacific Ocean.

Today, she just couldn't bear it. Her stomach turned at the turkey smell and she quietly collected the contents of her bag, ready to spring forth out the door before anyone could detain her to insist she take one of these cursed boxes, or pepper her with additional personal questions, or ask why she didn't smile more.

During the thirty seconds of polite applause at the end, Maggie bounded out of her chair and gave a wave and a head nod to DoCTR Debbie, hoping to suggest an urgency to get somewhere specific rather than to just escape in general. She kept it up until she was safely out the door and around the corner.

"Remember," the suit called after her as she darted out, "Computer Lab in an hour for modules! Don't be —" and the door shut behind Maggie before she could catch the last word.

As she race-walked away from the DoCTR, Maggie ran her hand along the wall, stopping when she reached Al's monstrous too-large face at the elevator, its eyes as big as lemons. *I'm dead, you know,* the face said silently as it smiled. Next to it, Marcus' face looked hopefully off into a bright future. *Al's dead,* it said to her. *Sellout,* she said in return, an insult the face reflected right back at her. She kept going past the elevator to the steel door leading into the stairwell. Her feet were itching to run (a feeling she almost never had). Her deconditioned heart, resigned to the task, chose *down* as the direction to take her, loose Danksos flopping off the ends of her feet as she went. *Kerthunk, kerthunk, kerthunk.* Wheezing with the effort, she eventually arrived at a door that said EXIT in large red letters and pushed through it. On the other side, she found herself on a familiar perch, a small concrete landing that looked out to a forested stretch of hillside.

Yes, she thought with relief, *YES.*

She hadn't consciously known this was where she was headed, but it was no accident. A worn opening headed into the underbrush, and Maggie followed it, a desire path she'd first become acquainted with ten years ago. About ten yards out, she came upon a clearing in the brush into which a metal folding chair and a large coffee can had been placed. There was a laminated NO SMOKING sign nailed onto one of the trees, but someone had crossed out the NO and replaced it with YES in black sharpie.

Yes, Maggie reflected back, pulling her smoking jacket out and zipping it up to the neck before lighting a smoke. She inhaled and felt the head-clearing endorphin burst of nicotine. As she exhaled, she unexpectedly began to cry.

She wasn't sure what she'd thought would come of her return. It had felt, when she pictured it in her mind, like the shiny glass buildings and the better pay and the waterfront condo views high above the city might somehow transport her out of her misery and into some new life, untouched by the pain of what had come before. That was foolish, of course, because pain can only live inside a person, and thus she *was* the pain, and could no sooner escape the pain as she could escape her own self, a feat she'd failed at again and again and again throughout her adult life. On the other hand, all else being equal, the pain might as well be experienced here, with more pain-money in a better pain-condo, where she could smoke as many pain-cigarettes as she liked and be free of the constant reminder of Christopher and his teflon perfection.

Had she also come here for Al? Perhaps. Was Al dead? Perhaps, again. Was this a dream? Maggie curled her toes in her shoes, feeling the smooth leather of the insole. She rubbed her eyes to the point of pain and opened them to find the same forest. She inhaled deeply again, holding the smoke in as long as she could muster before coughing it back out.

Before she knew it, her phone was open to the last messages with Al. Her own goofy face stared back at her from the photo she'd sent that morning, out of focus in favor of capturing the firetruck in the background. She scrolled back a bit to the message from three months ago, with the thumbs up, and then back before that to six months ago, the last day she'd seen Al in person. *Headed to the airport, talk soon?*

It hadn't received a response at the time, which had been its own kind of response. Maggie shivered and went back further, through a string of intermittent banter that had popped up in fits and spurts through the years. *Hey friend, hope you're taking it sleazy out in Missouri.* No real content, just light jabs and jives. *You know I am. I learned it from watching you.* Once a year, in the early fall, she'd send Al a photo of some kind of triangle (architectural, musical, Bermuda and the like) and receive back a volcano (Vesuvius, St. Helens, papier mâché with baking soda and vinegar) to commemorate an inside joke. She scrolled forward through several years of contact that had only been those photos, in different iterations, until she came to a message she'd sent a few years ago. *I'll be in town next week, wanna meet up?* Al had responded, *Name the time and place, I'm there.* Preserved in modern-day amber, as if scientists could resurrect her from the digital DNA to terrorize their island once more.

She looked at the little telephone handset icon at the top of the screen. *Push me,* it seemed to say, and Maggie obeyed. *Can't hurt, right?*

Ring, the phone responded as it presumptuously claimed to be calling *Al Power,* wherever she was on earth or in heaven or elsewhere.

Maggie held the phone up to her ear to listen, not really sure what she was expecting, but definitely not expecting to hear what she did after the second ring, which was Al's voice.

Al's voicemail hadn't changed since medical school. *You know who you reached, or you wouldn't be calling.* A knowing swagger in the delivery. *Throw some digits down after the beep and I'll hit you back.* Maggie smiled, hung up the phone, and tried to imagine the Medical Board calling that number repeatedly, leaving stern messages about drug screens and missed rehab meetings after the beep, Al contemplating how best to hit them back.

Was the voicemail evidence of Al's continued existence? Alternately, was there just an autopay still active from an abandoned account, paying and paying and paying to provide phone service to a dead woman? Was the primary function of the phone then to shuttle electronic money from one robot to another, so that a third robot could receive incoming calls largely from fourth and fifth and sixth and seventh robots whose duties were to place automated calls and leave messages about cable service and car warranties? Could these robots continue calling each other in Al's name until the end of time, should they please? Would this, then, make Al immortal?

As her wheels spun on this axle, something struck her (a thought, not an object), and she suddenly puffed out all the air from her lungs at once in surprise, air she hadn't realized was held in until it was suddenly out.

Two rings. *Two.* The phone had rung *two* times before going to voicemail. Not *four* rings, the voicemail number of rings. Maggie, admittedly, had left very few voicemails for very few people in the last few years, but surely *two* would not be the terminal ring number.

She pushed the telephone icon again, not really sure what theory she was testing, but knowing more data was required. *Ring.* Pause. *You know who you reached, or you wouldn't be calling.*

One ring, now? Maggie didn't for a second consider leaving a voicemail; never good at improv. Instead, she hung up and paced around the clearing, feet itching for action, one hand running through her ponytail while the other clutched the phone. She was losing her cool in a way that Frank T. Blood, Private Eye, would have found shameful.

Okay Frank, Maggie spoke to the specter of him that still sometimes lived in her head, *what do I do now?* Frank T. Blood was a man who always knew the next step, and she sometimes called upon him in moments like these. *C'mon Frank, I need ideas,* she said quietly.

Alice ain't dead, ma'am, Maggie heard a voice say from deep in the thicket surrounding her, *she's just hidin'.*

Was it a voice? It certainly sounded like a voice, but it had a static quality, like something not quite in full resolution, a radio signal being broadcast from the other side of the hill. But it *was* a voice, and the voice was weathered and deep, with the sandpaper veneer of a decades-old smoking habit, and the confidence of a white American man of a certain age. As Maggie looked out into the woods for a source, the voice laughed, a confident and bellied cackle that echoed off the side of the hospital building in surround sound. It was Frank's voice. Frank T. Blood, Private Eye.

I would sure know if she were dead, wouldn't I? Lord knows I can recognize the smell, the voice said. And he laughed again, a laugh that eventually devolved into a wet fit of coughing.

What are five things you can see, Maggie's therapist interjected. *What are five things you can hear?* Maggie swatted her hand in the air, uninterested in dropping anchor just yet.

On the one hand, Maggie knew Frank's voice was being generated in her mind's eye, and that she ought not traipse through the woods looking for the actual Frank T. Blood, who was, of course, long dead and cremated. On the other hand, Maggie was certain she had actually heard this voice with her actual ears. It was more than just a thought she had. It was a compression and release of the air around her, causing her tympanic membrane to vibrate, sending electrical impulses back to her auditory cortex. She knew this to be true, the same as she knew Frank to be dead.

Alice ain't dead, she's just hidin', Frank repeated.

A doctor is sort of like a scientist, and sort of like a priest. A doctor believes in an order of things, in mechanisms and enzymes and pharmacology and thermodynamics. A doctor also believes in luck and magic, in death that comes in threes and the dangers of being too nice or laboring under a full moon. In this moment, Maggie didn't entertain the possibility that this voice could be an acquired pathology. In this moment, Maggie found Frank's voice the same way some Catholics find St. Christopher or Buddhists find enlightenment. Maggie, who had once wished she could find God, had found Frank instead.

Alice ain't dead, she's just hidin', Frank repeated.

"Alright, Frank. Alright." She said this aloud, in her full voice. "What next?"

Before Frank could answer, Maggie's watch buzzed with a text notification from someone identifying themselves as DoCTR Debbie, reminding Maggie she was overdue back in the computer lab for module completion.

Hope you're on your way! Just a reminder! The modules are required before your first shift!

The chipper and exclamatory threats of a Suit, unmistakable.

Maggie's fist clenched, and she considered for a moment what it would be like to punch a tree, but thought better. *OK DoCTR Debbie,* she thought, *I'll play your game for now.*

"C'mon, Frank," Maggie said, throwing her burned-out cigarette in the coffee can, and heading back into the building. "We've got work to do."

The smoking jacket came off, but she didn't bother with the deodorant spray this time. She smelled her fingers and smiled, and walked back through the door.

Giddy-up, said Frank, *We've got work to do.*

Maggie arrived at the computer lab to find DoCTR Debbie standing at the door, repeatedly checking her watch. When she spotted Maggie, she mouthed *you made it* in a just-barely-audible whisper, smiling a seething and pointed smile. She gestured to a sign-in sheet on the table next to her. Maggie picked up the pen and paused over the blank space next to her name.

The fuck is this for, Frank asked over Maggie's shoulder, causing her to glance back. Frank leaned now against the door frame, fedora pulled low over his partially dissected forehead to cover up the absence of his *frontalis* muscle.

Did Maggie see this? She did see it. She blinked and rubbed her eyes, and Frank did the same right back at her.

You got a problem, he said, and Maggie didn't know if he was asking a question or making a statement. DoCTR Debbie tapped her finger on the sign-in sheet and cleared her throat, snapping Maggie's attention back to the task at hand.

The fuck is this for, Maggie thought, looking at the paper. Would this paper go into an accordion folder of sign-in-sheets that by regulation must be kept for seven years in a dusty basement storage room? Was there a sign-in-sheet storage technician? If the sign-in sheet were retired, would the job of the sign-in-sheet storage technician retire with it? Was the signing of the sheet then a humanitarian effort on Maggie's part?

Maggie looked up at DoCTR Debbie and smiled, then looked down and wrote *Frank T. Blood* in dramatic, looping cursive next to her own name. *Perhaps the sign-in-sheet technician will get a kick out of this.*

Maggie found a computer along a side wall, as far from Debbie's gaze as she could manage where she could exert minimal effort with maximal distraction. These onboarding modules always took the same form, timed slides you can't advance through, a quiz at the end, but anyone who has taken these quizzes enough times would know the questions are always softballs lobbed up to weed out only the functionally illiterate. *If you suspect Medicare Fraud, should you a) call the Medicare Fraud hotline, b) tell your mom, c) post it on SocialEyes.* When your job is to write the quizzes for regulatory compliance modules, lord knows you need to find humor somewhere. *What should you do after removing gloves that are soiled with blood? a) eat lunch, b) pick your nose, c) wash or sanitize your hands.*

It was as if the quiz-writers, locked in the same thankless system of nonsense as everyone else, were reaching out to say, *we are human, too. We have families. Please pass this quiz and we can all go home, okay?* The system is not here for you. The system is not here for me. The system is here for itself.

Maggie put on the headphones, logged in, and got to clicking. The clicking was hypnotic, soothing, meditative, like when she was tasked with repeating the Hail Mary over and over again as a kid when she'd done something wrong. What was she doing penance for now? Something, surely. Like all doctors, touched by an original sin she could never truly atone for. Click, click. *Hail Medicare, full of grace.* What are the five types of PHI? *The wards are with thee.* Click, click. What are the four steps to use a fire extinguisher? *Blessed art thou among regulators, and blessed is the fruit of thy womb, The Joint Commission, JC Christ.* Click, click. Does the P in PASS stand for a) Pull, b) Pneumonia, or c) Pterodactyl? *Holy Medicare, Preventer of Fraud, pray for us doctors, now and in the hour of our death.* Each click moving another regulatory rosary bead one stop down the line. Click. Click. Click. *Amen.*

The final module was entitled "Survival in an Active Shooter Situation," and for a moment, Maggie stopped clicking and looked away.

Not this bullshit, said Frank in her ear, laughing and laughing and laughing and laughing, in that manic way that people laugh at unfunny things. *Who needs to survive anyway?*

Maggie looked for a mute button on the screen, finding it to be grayed out. She sighed loudly, pointedly, and imagined herself as a cloud, vaporizing in the chair, losing her substance and floating through the air vents and out of the building. In this gaseous form, she slipped the headphones just off the back of her ears, reducing the intensity of their output, but not the fact of it. As the video auto-played, the head of hospital security came on screen to say: *Thousands of people have survived active shooting situations, and you can too.*

Had he been instructed to focus on the positives in his talk? *We want it to be uplifting,* some hospital exec had probably told the man, *to build resilience.* Maggie floated above the building like a gaseous, translucent god.

Run, hide, fight, the man said as he cataloged all the routes of egress and hiding places in the hospital *in the event of hostile activity,* speaking around the specifics of this *hostile activity* in the way people do to soften the blows of death and violence. *Run, indeed,* Maggie thought, as she opened up another browser window to at least hide the active-shooter re-enactment from her non-consenting eyes.

Watch as these nurses pass by the elevator to seek egress through a staff-only stairwell. They will survive this, because they have planned for it. In the absence of safety, we have procedures. If the procedures make you *feel* safe, isn't that as good as the safety itself?

No running or hiding for me, said Frank into Maggie's ear. *Not for Frank T. Blood, no ma'am. Frank T. Blood* faces *his enemies.*

Good for you, Frank, Maggie said back to him silently, as she typed *causes of visual hallucinations* into Google. Her eyes skipped right over *Schizophrenia* and *Drug-Induced Psychosis* and landed on *Charles Bonnet Syndrome,* which sounded more poetic, and therefore, acceptable. *Charles Bonnet Syndrome refers to the phenomenon of visual hallucinations that occur after significant vision loss.* Perhaps she wasn't going crazy, perhaps she was just going blind. *Anton's Syndrome,* she continued reading, *refers to the condition when a person with cortical blindness denies the fact of their vision loss.* Perhaps she was both crazy *and* blind. Perhaps none of this was real at all.

The security guy was cataloging the items in a hospital that could be used as weapons in a pinch. *An IV pole. A cautery pen. Try not to find yourself engaging in hand to hand combat if you can help it, but if it isn't avoidable, a fire extinguisher can act as both a smokescreen and a battering ram. IV tubing is quite strong and can be used to restrain a perpetrator if you manage to subdue him.*

Maggie rubbed her eyes again, vision working totally fine, as far as she could tell. Before she could stop her fingers, she had abandoned Google and moved on to SocialEyes. In a world where nursing staff were expected to know guerrilla warfare countermeasures, so what if SocialEyes was a Russian asset designed for election interference? *If you're going to tie hospital bed sheets together to egress from a higher floor, be sure to make a square knot to avoid slippage.* So what if some guy makes incrementally more billions of dollars because of your eyeballs on his content? *A good rule of thumb is that it takes three hospital bed sheets for each floor of the hospital.* So. What.

She tested her old login on a hunch. Could she remember her password even? *1234SocialEyespassword*, she typed, and then she was in.

It had been an overstatement when Maggie claimed to have deleted SocialEyes. The deletion had been passive and internal, a deletion that had only occurred within her own heart. The app was removed from her smartphone, sure. The links removed from her browser, yes. But nothing was really *deleted,* just left in stasis. Today, it awoke happily to her prodigal return. The messaging icon in the corner flagged 72, suggesting that a number of people in her life had not gotten the messages she hadn't sent them about deleting Social-Eyes. It had waited for her, like an ex-boyfriend in the parking lot. Like a rattlesnake around the corner of the trail. Like a spider in a shoe. *She'll be back eventually,* it had correctly predicted.

The top post on her feed was from one of her female classmates, now a cardiothoracic surgeon, who apparently just had a baby. *Introducing Helen Marie! We are so over the moon,* the caption said, followed by three different moon emojis and a picture of a hospital-gowned woman holding a newborn. The baby's head was perfectly round, which Maggie knew meant a C-section birth. Her classmate's face was glassy-eyed, pale, with a wan smile that toed a line between forced and genuine. *Probably IVF,* Maggie thought, knowing this classmate to be almost certainly in her mid-40s at least, knowing how Maggie's own reproduction had been delayed until the statistical chance of a happy and healthy outcome was below a certain threshold, and eventually how she had realized that remaining *#childfree* was a choice she had made rather than a product of her circumstance.

Christopher had intermittently brought up *seeing a specialist* or *just talking to the adoption agency, no pressure,* but Maggie had deferred and delayed for the time not being quite right, and *let's just wait until respiratory season is over* became *maybe when I'm not working night shifts anymore* became *maybe let's just see what the outcome of the election is,* until eventually it became an appointment to have a 10-year IUD placed and that was that. When she had gone to her gynecologist, she had been handed a marketing brochure for the IUD. On the cover there was a photo of a woman pushing a swing, except in the swing, instead of a human child, was a high-end camera on a tripod. *THIS IS MY BABY, NOW,* said the tagline under the photo, and Maggie laughed, thinking of what she would be putting into her own swing.

This is my baby now, as Maggie pushes around a pack of cigarettes in a stroller. *This is my baby now,* as she zips up the onesie of her clinical depression. *This is my baby now,* as she changes the diaper on her stalled, pathetic medical career. Unrelatedly, this was around the time she and Christopher had stopped having sex altogether, and the poor IUD had since stood stalwart protecting a gate at which no one was knocking, hardly to be battle-tested at all.

What's the use of procreating in a world that won't last their life expectancy anyhow, Maggie thought, cruelly, as she looked at the smiling face of her classmate and her angelic babe. She continued to scroll through the home page as the training video had moved on to describing methods for creating effective barricades in defensible spaces. *Titanium orthopedic implants can be used to bar the doors of an OR. A mobile fluoroscopy machine is heavy and CAN be an effective blockade, but you have to remember to chalk the wheels.*

SocialEyes was offering a different kind of blockade. Old classmates' family updates. Surgical techs from Missouri selling leggings and body wraps. Handgun memes from distant cousins in Texas. Interpolated with these, Simone Biles highlight reels, blooper videos from *The Office,* videos about tracking ovulatory cycles, advertisements for supplements meant to boost fertility, videos of dogs doing that cute thing with their head where it tilts to one side. Videos that, before she had joined the *#deleteSocialEyes* revolution, she had fallen asleep to night after night after night, lying in bed with her phone as Christopher snored gently beside her. Had her life been better for their absence these last seven years? It would be hard to argue the point.

She found herself lingering on the videos now as she did then. Unable to scroll past a highlight of Simone Biles' triumphant beam routine from the Tokyo Olympics until she had seen it to a stuck-landing completion. Unable to resist the follow-up reel of gymnastics bloopers that autoplayed after it was done. Unable to stop as Social-Eyes took her on a ride into '*Gymnastics Disasters!!!*', videos of young, mostly Eastern European women in the 1980s landing awkwardly on their necks in international competition. These gruesome videos made her feel a mixture of sadness and horror, but she continued to watch anyhow.

Jesus Christ, what're you dickin' around for, doc? Frank said. *Get to it.*

Maggie closed her eyes as a young Russian gymnast hobbled around the floor exercise after suffering a brain stem injury on a now-banned salto move. Her eyes opened, and she reluctantly navigated to the search field and typed in *Alice Power.* Was that what Frank wanted?

Now we're talking, said Frank.

The top result was a post by their class president Elizabeth three months ago, that read as follows:

Hey guys. I am sorry to report some bad news.
I received word today from Alice Power's brother that she lost her battle
with alcohol last week.
The family requests privacy at this time.

That ain't no obituary, Frank said, *that's your first clue.* Maggie could hear him puffing away at a cigarette while he spoke. *You know who requests privacy,* he added, *people with somethin' to HIDE.*

The security guy in the module was wrapping up. *We are living in unprecedented times,* he was saying, *but you can be a survivor.* Maggie blinked her eyes quickly three times, as if to break a spell. She closed the SocialEyes browser, leaving Alice's death announcement and the maimed and tragic gymnasts and the 72 messages behind. A quiz was waiting for her in the other browser.

What is the best option if faced with an active shooter situation?

a) Run, b) Play Dead, c) Try to convert the shooter to Quakerism.

This is the system that maintains a doctor. She was a doctor, wasn't she still? Maggie got 100% on the quiz, closed the browser, and in one motion gathered her belongings, pushed her chair back, and sprung again out the door before DoCTR Debbie could argue otherwise.

Chapter 4

MS1

Back in the dissection lab, it was Friday of their first week, and the group had been working together long enough to have relaxed into a familiar banter that distracted them from the oddity of the work itself. "Do they make serrated scalpels?" Christopher mused, working his way through a particularly beefy length of *longissimus dorsi* as Maggie looked on. "It feels like I need a steak knife for this thing." He was hunched over, sweating, the tallest at a table that had not been calibrated for his height.

"Dude, your scalpel blade is just dull. You gotta get a new one," Al replied as she worked from the other side of the table. "Replace it every day, man, it should go through *like butter.*" She pronounced this last word with an exaggerated east coast flare, *like buttah*, and everyone laughed.

"A new blade every day? That feels like such a waste, you know?" Christopher held up the scalpel blade. "Did you know they burn these in incinerators after we're done? Medical waste is so insane."

Al was incredulous. "Why are you worried about a little scalpel blade? You know all these *bodies* are gonna get cremated, too. Why bother?"

Christopher paid no mind to this statement, turning the blade over in his fingers to examine the structure. "Maybe I'll bring a leather strop tomorrow so we can just sharpen them. That's probably allowed, right?"

Maggie looked over at him and smiled, pulling her attention briefly away from the *erector spinae* muscle she had been delineating with her own (sharp, fresh) scalpel blade.

"What a great idea, Christopher. Very thoughtful," Maggie replied, because a midwestern woman is encouraging, after all.

"Yes," added Al with a smile. "How *very* thoughtful." Al caught Maggie's eye from across the table, and Maggie blushed. Maggie and Christopher had, mostly by default, ended up working together on the body's left side, while Al and Jess worked together on the right, a configuration that had just stuck from day one. The arrangement set Maggie up perfectly to take periodic cross-table glances at Al, glances she wasn't sure why she made, except that Al just seemed to command attention in that way. Working as they did in a mirror image of one another across Frank's body, Al seemed like a funhouse reflection of what Maggie might have looked like if she were different in every possible way but living the same life.

"Speaking of steak knives and butter, don't you just crave a good steak after dissection lab?" Al had just released a long section of back muscle that did, for all intents and purposes, look just like an over-cooked tenderloin. She looked over her shoulder to confirm the absence of any nearby authorities and lowered her voice. "I mean, doesn't this look like it needs a good sear and an *au jus?*"

"Good god, Alice, is that necessary? I'm already a vegetarian," said Christopher. "Now more than ever."

"Dude, I haven't been able to eat meat since we started," Jess agreed. "And I may never be able to again, thanks to you. Well, you and *the smell.*"

The smell.

The smell was the uncreative name they had given for the partic-ular *eau de parfum* that had emanated from Frank T. Blood since the first incision on day one. *The smell* had grown, slowly and surely, more potent and noxious with each uncovered layer and each passing day.

Frank, it seemed, had been preserved in haste (or perhaps not preserved at all, they were even starting to suspect). Maggie would stroll by the other bodies on her way back to the corner, inhaling surreptitiously as she passed, and had noted that none of the other cadavers seemed to be quite as. . .*ripe*. The other bodies were serene and plasticine and inert, whereas Frank was anything but. Rather than being arrested in stasis, Frank's body seemed to *change* from day to day. The muscle bodies would be red and meaty when first uncovered, and then would turn brown, and then gray as a day or two passed. Worst of all, Frank's initially concave abdomen had been slowly moving toward convexity with the forces of what seemed like gaseous distention, a bloating force that was slowly lifting his still-prone body up just so slightly off of the table, like a balloon inflating in slow motion at the Macy's Day Parade. Now five days in, his body had started to tilt at an awkward angle on the table with the upward forces of it, and the group were being careful not to exert too much *downward* pressure so as to force the release of whatever it was that was trapped within.

And the smell. *The Smell.* The group was locked fiercely in a chemical arms race with it as their wimpy Vicks Vap-O-Rub had been thoroughly outgunned on day one. *The Smell* had subsequently bested both peppermint and tea tree oils, and was now working head to head against N95 respirators lined with lavender and cedar extracts (an idea brought to the table after the team had spent a night investigating Egyptian mummification protocols). This was working well enough to keep dry heaving at bay, though Christopher had scored some Zofran tablets that were kept in his back pocket, just in case. For good measure, they had several open boxes of baking soda standing around the table, probably doing nothing from a strictly scientific perspective, but maybe providing some sort of spiritual protection anyhow. They had not yet ruled out the principles of witchcraft and/or Catholic exorcism to manage the situation, being less than a week deep into eleven weeks of co-existence with The Smell. *You never know.* There was sage in Jess' locker and a large container of salt as well. *It can't hurt.* Medicine is 90% science, but the remaining 10% is pure and unapologetic superstition. Death comes in threes. Babies are born with the full moon. Don't say the Q word. Sprinkle salt around the cadaver, why not. *It can't hurt.*

On day 2, Dr. Bald Man had stopped by on his daily rounds as the group worked in misery, and Maggie had felt a wave of relief. Surely, *surely* this professional cadaver-man would have some way to rectify the situation, if he only knew about The Smell. Perhaps a replacement body? A second dose of formaldehyde? Dr. Bald Man (not his real name) had sidled up next to Jess and put his hand on the middle of her back in a way that made her muscles tighten, but that she didn't audibly object to. He rested a hip against the table and laughed on arrival, waving his free hand in front of his nose in the universal sign of *something stinks*, and his body had shaken itself up and down against the edge of the table in a way that made Frank T. Blood rock gently back and forth on his own bulbous abdomen. "Hm, looks like you guys got a ripe one!" Dr. Bald Man had said, patting Jess on the back as she looked across the table at Maggie with wide eyes. "Well, there's always one in the room!" He patted again and laughed again. "Whew! Well, good luck!" Another laugh, another table shake. Then he walked away.

With that, hope had been lost. There would be no rapture out of this purgatory. No exchange for a new specimen. No additional formaldehyde treatment. No apologies. No *help*. Even the surgical residents, otherwise immune to most corporeal insults, just avoided their group and their smell altogether, focusing their teaching efforts as far across the room as possible. Perhaps it was Maggie's imagination, but it also seemed to her that all the other tables were slowly drifting away from them, as if to maroon them on an island of their own misery, mirroring the heat death of the universe.

The system is here to produce doctors, and it was producing doctors, wasn't it? So the system is working. The system is not here to *help* you. The system is here to *mold* you. So there they were, on day five, in the midst of this system and its smell, Al making jokes about steaks, the rest of the group swearing off meat, five days closer to being doctors.

"I was trying to do keto before school started, can you believe that?" Jess said, patting her flat midsection as she said this. "*That* didn't last long. This is like *all* carbs right here." Jess had multiple buffering folds of fabric between her and any hint of what was happening with her body, but a sharp shadow below her cheekbones suggested that an excess of carbohydrate was not the issue at hand.

"I guess I can sympathize a little bit with cannibal societies," Maggie said, taking in the look of the *multifidus* muscle body that she was carving away from its facet joints below. "We are kind of made outta meat, you know? No different from a cow or a chicken." Jess wrinkled her nose and mimed backing away slowly from Maggie.

"Jeez! Nobody accept a dinner invitation from you, amirite?" The group laughed, and Al laughed a deep and fundamental laugh, and looked into Maggie's eyes when she did, so Maggie doubled down.

"I'm just *saying*, like, if you were *starving* somewhere, wouldn't you?"

Al's eyes were locked on Maggie.

"Oh, you *know* I would, Maggie. You know I would." In spite of the icy blue of Al's eyes, Maggie felt the slightest bit of heat, and suddenly she felt like a different version of herself.

Jess eyed Maggie and Al with suspicion. "Just so you know, I am *not* made of meat. I am made of rainbows and fairy dust. So don't get any ideas." Jess brushed her shoulders off as she spoke, and gave Maggie a little smile.

"Naw, you're made of meat," said Al. "Meat!" She held up another portion of muscle to make her point. "*Meat.*"

"Did you know humans are made of the same stuff as stars? The very same," said Christopher, who was back to hacking away with a dull blade, shredding to pieces the muscle he was meant to be removing *en bloc*, but damned if he was going to give in to a new scalpel blade *now*.

"Sorry," said Maggie. "I almost forgot we were in the House of God." She looked up at Al, who had passed a copy of the book *The House of God* to her a few days prior.

"House of God's played out. We're stuck in The House of *Gas*," said Al, poking gingerly at the out-pouching of Frank's distending belly. "Hey, do you guys play any instruments? Because *Frank T. Blood and the Gas* isn't a bad name for a band. I'll be the lead singer, of course." Al threw the hunk of muscle she'd been holding into a bucket under the table labeled DISCARD.

"I can play the flute?" said Maggie, apologetically.

"I play a little guitar myself," said Christopher.

"I can take tambourine," said Jess.

"It's settled, then. We've got ourselves a band!"

Al started singing an imagined first track as she continued to throw little bits of Frank into the bucket. "*We're all made of meeeeeat. Me and you and Frank T. Bloooood. We're all made of meeeeat. We start as meat! We live as meat! And theeeeen weeeeee Die! As! Meat!*"

Maggie tried to whistle a melodic flute line as Al continued: "*Made of meat (meat, meat), Made of meat (meat, meat), I never met a man with stinkier feet, then Frankie Bloooooooood . . .*"

Al paused here to catch her breath, and Christopher half-heartedly added a guitar solo.

"*. . .and his big old bags of meeeeeeeeat!*"

"Not bad for our first rehearsal," said Maggie encouragingly.

For the rest of the day, Alice and Maggie and Jess and Christopher sang little ditties about Frank as they passed the time, imagining themselves as rock stars who were taking a break from their European tour in this anatomy lab.

"*Frankieeeee, Fraaaaaaankie, he's a man with a plaaaaaan. He ain't got skin but he's got two hands, and he'll never be lonely agaaaaaaain,*" sang Al, perfectly on key.

"*Mr. Blood, you're a bad bad man, with a smell so bad you won't eeeeeever make, anooooootheeeer frieeeeend,*" sang Maggie, not on key at all.

Frank T. Blood laid still as he took this abuse, face shrouded, hands flopping uselessly by his sides.

As his sinew was torn asunder, Frank's body told a kind of story about Frank's past life. Frank's body was younger than the other cadavers, the group had deduced, as the muscles had not yet undergone the fatty atrophy of old age. The other bodies, broadly speaking, told the stories of erudite elder ladies and learned old men who had lived through many golden years and had made estate donations to their alma maters along with their bodies. Frank's body sang a different tune. No, this body did not tell the story of a long farewell, did not tell of post-retirement ease, did not tell of a rocking chair and watching sunsets and sipping tea and lazy afternoon naps. Frank's body spoke of toil and lifting and action and sweat that had abruptly ended at the peak of its power. Frank's life had cultivated a sinew so firm and taut and ready as to require speculation about the need for serrated scalpels.

And yet. . .somehow, the man laid here prone and helpless while medical students (weak and pale, the lot of them) flayed him open and argued about the relative similarities of his muscles to cuts of steak, muscles that would never chop wood or climb a barbed wire fence or restrain a fleeing bounty ever again.

How had he come to pass? Their clipboard said only, *Unknown Natural Cause*. What could that mean for a man this age, other than no one had cared enough to find out? Overdose? Aneurysm? Apoplexy? At some point, a medical examiner had rolled up to this body, found by paramedics or police perhaps, lifeless and alone. Maybe it was the middle of the night, and the medical examiner hadn't slept a full night in a week owing to a string of opioid overdoses downtown, and he had simply shrugged his shoulders and said, "Yeah, looks like a man who was meant to die young," and moved on. *Not all mysteries need to be solved,* he might have muttered under his breath, a fact a seasoned doctor knows all too well, but medical students (still believing in an orderly and logical world) can have a hard time accepting.

These particular medical students, at least, were not yet at that place of acceptance.

Leukemia, Alice postulated, having noticed a paucity of fat reserves, maybe a sign of some overly active metabolic state that had consumed Frank's energy too fast for him to keep up. *Something that took him quickly, but not totally without warning.* Blood cancer was a convenient theory since it couldn't be disproved; his blood having been drained and replaced by formaldehyde and long since discarded into a big red bag marked as *Biohazard* and sent to an incinerator. *Sepsis,* Maggie had suggested, *overwhelming infection. Based on the smell.*

The smell.

The smell was its own mystery and brought with it both a sense of urgency and nihilism to the group. On one hand, *I can't wait to get out of here today.* On the other, *what does it matter when we have to come back tomorrow?* Pain can be a motivator, though, and it had been for Maggie, who was spending her evenings poring over the dissection manual to work as efficiently as possible. Today, Maggie had been ready for what the next page on the dissection manual revealed.

"A saw?" Jess exclaimed when she read it. "A *saw?*"

"Yeah," Al said. "How else did you think surgeons get into the spinal cord? Fairy dust and wishes?"

"Thank god I'm going to be a dermatologist," Jess said. "Surgery is gross."

Jess didn't know this then, but even a dermatologist would not be spared the grotesquerie of the human condition. Eventually, Jess will have to (for instance) contend with the necrotic reality of advanced squamous cell carcinoma and its tendency to attract maggots (yes, *actual maggots*). Eventually, Jess will live in a world where the most famous member of her profession will be an internet celebrity who squeezes pimples on camera. No one in medicine escapes the vulgarities of human frailty, not even a dermatologist. But today, of this, Jess remained blissfully unaware, and stood back from the table with her arms crossed.

Christopher offered to do the deed, owing to his prior experience with power tools and all."Seems like this'll be right up my alley as a Midwesterner, right?" He spoke with a twangy affectation for effect, and had already picked up the saw.

"Actually, I think Maggie should do it," Al interjected, looking intently at Maggie. She timed this perfectly, catching both Christopher and Maggie off guard. "She's Midwestern too, right? She looks like she can handle a bone saw."

Maggie wasn't sure if this was a compliment or not, but she

blushed as if it were, and did not object. Her forehead started to sweat with a performance anxiety she hadn't tapped into since a sixth-grade piano recital, but she tried to play it cool.

"Yeah, I know my way around a power tool," Maggie said with borrowed confidence.

Christopher ceded the saw to her, showing her how to operate the foot switch as Maggie donned safety glasses. Maggie liked the heft of the saw in her hand; the way holding it made her bicep pop out just a little bit. She pointed at the vertebrae she planned to cut, like Babe Ruth calling his shot before stepping up to the plate.

"Here, right?"

Maggie had looked up at Al as she said this, and Al looked directly back at her. Under the punishing overhead track-lighting, Al's eyes were a near-fluorescent blue, like two ancient icebergs that had found their way onto Al's otherwise dark features. One of those icebergs winked at Maggie and said, "Don't ask me, you're the one holding the saw."

Maggie was thankful for the presence of her mask in this moment to obscure her flushed cheeks. The icebergs were certainly used to getting this response from people, Maggie thought, before turning back to the bone and the task at hand.

The squeal of the saw motor filled her ears, and she focused her mind as she tilted it down onto the bone and braced her hands against the vibration. She recited the layers of the spinal canal in her mind as she worked through the bone, one millimeter at a time, worried about bagging the dorsal root ganglion or busting through the bone too harshly and severing the spinal cord.

Ligamentum Flavum. Yellow ligament, she thought, remembering her Latin roots. *Dura mater. Arachnoid mater. Pia mater.* Small bits of aerosolized bone were flung against her safety glasses, putting her view into a softer focus. She worked slowly, using her internal recitation as a kind of countdown. *Thick mother, spider mother, tender mother,* she thought. *Dura mater, Arachnoid mater, Pia mater.* She moved from the left side to the right side. What are these mothers doing behind this bony door? The thick mother, the spider mother, and the tender mother, like characters in a nursery rhyme. The tender mother holds the spinal cord so closely that you'd be hard pressed to separate it from the cord itself, except for the delicate tendrils of the mother that spin out and attach the cord to bone. These attachments keep the cord from spinning and twisting in the fluid environment of the spinal canal, like tender mother shackles inside a tender mother prison. It's for the cord's own good, of course.

The bone gave way, and Maggie lifted out the saw, holding it with her elbow cocked up next to her ear, like a shotgun.

"We're in," she said, as if she'd just cracked a safe. "We're *in*." She lifted out the spinous process and held it tenderly like a treasure in her outstretched hands. Revealed beneath the now-absent bone was a glistening butter-yellow layer of *dura mater.*

"Hello, mother," Maggie said under her breath.

Al gave a little *woot, woot* of encouragement.

Christopher gave Maggie a hearty pat on her shoulder. "Not bad, for, well. . ." He caught himself before he could finish that particular thought. "Not bad!"

Maybe it was the reflection of the over-bright fluorescent lights off of the snow-white bit of bone, maybe it was the adrenaline burst of saw operation that had dilated her pupils, but for a moment, though the 3rd sub-basement had no windows, Maggie could swear she felt the sun shining upon her face. For the first time since she arrived, a feeling crept into her that maybe, just maybe, she might belong here.

The system may be a one-way rocket ship shot into space, and you may be a dog in a space-suit strapped inside its doomed hull, but for a brief, magic moment, perhaps you will get to gaze upon the totality of the earth-at-once, and your walnut brain will fill with transcendent awe as you howl at the now-miles-closer moon. No need to worry about what comes next, in a moment like this.

This is the system that creates a doctor, after all, and in this moment, the system is absolutely perfect.

The next week passed with a series of similar triumphs. Maggie successfully isolated a hard-to-locate dorsal root ganglion. Maggie got a perfect score on the first test. Maggie was referred to as a *secret gunner* by one of her classmates, to which she'd replied, *"How can I be a gunner, I went to a state school,"* which was the only right answer. Maggie remained the official Bone Saw Operator of *Frank T. Blood and the Gas.*

On Day 11, Maggie and Jess stood in the women's locker room, peeling down to their bras and underwear. (Where was Al in this locker room? Somehow, Maggie had never seen her. It seemed she just *appeared* in the lab each day, as if by magic. Maggie knew better than to question it.) Maggie and Jess discussed the relative merits of Neutrogena T-Gel or Herbal Essences or Charcoal shampoo for removing odors from hair as they tied up scrub pants with ties that seemed to be getting longer and longer as their post-lab appetite had grown weaker and weaker, and their caffeine intake had gone up and up and up.

"Did you look ahead for the day?" Jess said after they were put together and shuffling out of the locker room.

"Oh, you know me," Maggie responded, tucking her shirt in as they walked, unfazed now at the thought of having her hand deep into the front of her pants in this hallway full of mixed company. "I couldn't sleep again last night, so I just studied instead."

"Frank in your dreams again?"

Maggie nodded. "I dreamed he was pregnant."

The dream, from which Maggie had awoken in a shock at three AM, involved the group uncovering a live fetus that had secretly been growing in Frank's lower intestine, living off of the necrotic fuel of his dissolving innards. Afraid to fall back asleep, Maggie had instead flipped through her Netter's Clinical Anatomy until the sun had come up. "I guess I should thank him if I end up with an honors grade," she said.

A midwestern woman knows better than to take credit for her own accomplishments.

Jess changed the subject. "Anything I need to know for today? I haven't looked at *anything* yet, I'm so far behind it's not even funny."

Jess often played this *who me study* routine that Maggie eventually would recognize as an act, especially since Jess would eventually match into Dermatology, which you can't do without an honors grade in Gross Anatomy; an honors grade that requires a thousand minutiae to have inserted themselves into your brain either through concerted effort or divine provenance. Jess knew the long game, though. Act casual, not like some kind of try-hard, just shrug and cast your eyes down when the test scores return and say something like *oh I guess I did alright haha*. A woman must not be boastful or crass. A woman must sneak into the halls of power through a side door.

"Jess." Maggie stopped in her tracks. "You *must* know what today is." Maggie wasn't smiling.

"Well — I don't *really* know, but I might be able to guess?" Jess kept walking, and Maggie was forced to keep up.

The day before, the group had been working their way down the landscape of Frank's backside, reaching the peaks of the gluteal region by the end of the day. They had learned satisfying words like *piriformis, pudendal, obturator*. However, the expedition had left (conspicuously, one might say) the more *ahem* midline structures unscathed. "I was sort of hoping we'd just move on down to hamstrings today."

"NOPE."

"Damn."

They arrived at their table and flipped their dissection guides in unison to the next page: 8.1 THE ANAL TRIANGLE, it said to them, menacingly.

Maggie looked over at Jess, who had a look on her face of either pain or suppressed laughter, or possibly both. The taut silence burst as a voice called from behind Maggie's shoulder. The voice was imitating a pirate, starting with a whisper and reaching a fevered crescendo near her ear.

"*Aye aye, matey! Be ye warned* whoever shall seek the treasure of the Anal Triangle, turn back, ye! YE SHALL NOT RETURN FROM ITS DEPTHS! CURSED BE ALL WHO SEEK ITS FECAL TREASURES!"

Maggie turned to find Al, pantomiming a pirate hook with one hand and limping on an imagined peg leg. Maggie instinctively held a finger up to her lips and looked around in equal parts embarrassment and delight. There was not a professor in sight, but still she felt (as all medical students do) that someone must at all times be watching and making notes for the permanent record. *Lacks professional decorum*, somewhere it might be written. *Relies on childish humor.*

"What's got into you Al? *Cut it out.*" Maggie's smile was making a different request, one that Al clocked perfectly.

"*KEEP YER HANDS OFF ME BOOTY, ARRRRrrrrrr,*" Al continued.

"Dude, Alice, knock it off. This is med school, not an improv troupe." Christopher had arrived to be a voice of reason. "You've had your fun." He rolled his eyes conspicuously and opened his dissection guide, coming to the same realization the rest of the group had a moment ago. "Aw, shit."

"*Exactly,*" said Al. "Just trying to break the ice before we break the *ass,* you know?" Al was relentless sometimes. Maggie had learned that pushing back was useless, even when it became tiresome.

"Well," said Christopher, "*you* want to be the surgeon, why don't you do the honors today. Since there's only one anal triangle, seems like it's a one man job."

"Well, I think you'd be surprised at how many men an anal triangle can accommodate." Alice had a serious face, dead serious, but her eyes were not serious.

Could you blame her? How can a person, faced with an anal triangle, a slowly bloating cadaver, the *booty* pun sitting right there for the taking, the daytime delirium that always follows sleepless study nights — how can a person maintain decorum at a time like this? These jokes will cross your mind no matter what you do, they might as well be voiced and released to dissipate this odorous miasma of misery for at least a moment.

"Dude, that's *enough.*" Christopher was standing up to his full imposing height, leaning just over the table. Al cast her iceberg eyes right back at him and crossed her arms across her chest, corners of her mouth angled just upward.

"Alright, man, alright. I guess no one likes Al's jokes but they like her knife skills, do I have that right? Should I just shut up and cut?"

Maggie did not like where this posturing was headed, in this delicate setting with a teetering gas-filled dead man sitting atop a table packed with drawers full of sharp knives.

"Hey, guys. I'll dissect today. Just chill." Maggie pulled on gloves (two pairs, for good measure), adjusted her mask, pinched the nose piece firmly to cut off nasal airflow, and practiced the reverse circular breathing that she had learned to do to minimize exposure to her sensitive olfactory nerves. "No reason to fight over it. Any job that needs doin' is worth being done by you. That's what my grandfather used to say." A midwestern woman does what needs doing, after all.

"Fuck yeah, Maggie!" Jess was vocally enthusiastic in her support, which she was providing from several feet away at the head of the bed, arms crossed.

Maggie looked over at Al. "Al, how about you navigate, I'll drive, okay?"

"Avast, into uncharted waters we sail," Al replied, looking at Christopher. Maggie rolled her eyes as she readied her scalpel.

"Don't make me laugh, I might end up inhaling through my nose."

"Aye-aye, captain," Al responded, her face showing Maggie there was more material she wasn't using, and everyone should be glad for her restraint.

Maggie and Al set sail, Maggie's confidence boosted by her recent success with the bone saw and by Al's soft encouragement as she went along. "This isn't so bad," Maggie said to Al as she delicately made the first 12:00 incision and used the flat edge of the scalpel to gently peel up a dermal edge.

"Not bad at all," Al agreed. "You're doing great. Remember, the muscle is just underneath here, so don't go too deep."

"I never have and I never will," said Maggie, using a hemostat to pinch the leading edge while her scalpel teased the superficial skin free from its underlying structures. This confident voice that had emerged after bone saw day was feeling more and more comfortable for Maggie. "C'mon, Frank. Nice and easy," Maggie spoke absent-mindedly as she worked. "Just come on off. You don't need this skin, do you? No, no you don't. Just come with me. There!"

"Maggie, are you talking to the anal sphincter?" Maggie's sweet talk had caught the attention of Jess, who had been watching from the head of the table. "I think you might be losing it."

Maggie paused her work for a moment and looked up at Jess with a furrowed brow. "You know Jess, at the end of the day, I'm just a girl, standing in front of a sphincter. . ." she paused, trying to think of a punchline, and couldn't.

Al jumped in. "Asking it to deglove for her?"

"God, you guys deserve each other," Jess said as she went back to flipping through flashcards. Maggie and Al carried on; Al looking on admiringly as Maggie pulled fat globules off the surface of the sphincter's burgundy dome. "Maggie, I must say, that is one fine-looking muscle."

"Technically, Alice, it is *three* muscles, working together." Maggie indicated to the dissection diagram that was propped up on what would have been the small of Frank's back, if it hadn't been taken down past the bone already. "Subcutaneous, superficial, and deep."

"Sounds like my first time," Al responded. Maggie ignored this, or perhaps didn't hear it in her bubble of concentration.

"Al, where do you think the nerve is gonna be?" Maggie was using a finger to probe around the fatty tissue, hoping to feel one of the fibrous strands or plump vessels there to mark it before cutting any deeper.

"Three-o-clock, I think. If you think of the coccyx as high noon and the balls as six."

On a human body, anything round is discussed in terms of a clock face. Anuses and breasts, keeping a type of time with their hemorrhoids and lumps.

"Testes, please, Al. Testes. Scrotum, even. But not balls. Balls are for gym class."

Al gave her a little salute. "Testes it is, m'lady."

Right in that moment, with Al's good humor upon her and this beautifully dissected (she didn't mind saying) sphincter muscle before her, Maggie had a clear and vivid thought: *this ain't half bad.* If that satisfaction was the feeling of being a doctor, she could get used to it. Maggie and Alice had their heads huddled together over the exposed anus as if it were a campfire keeping them warm, both of them searching through the yellow fat for the glimpse of a spark of white nerve, eyebrows furrowed and focused, olfactory inputs parked on a back burner somewhere in the throes of their concentration. Al started singing an impromptu sea shanty.

"Frankie was the privatest guuuuy, with haaaair of black and a brown winkiiiing eeeeye," Al sang, as Jess did a little jig in the background. Maggie, in that moment, was feeling self-assured, confident, in control, blissful even.

If you ever get this feeling, dear reader, take note, for this is the feeling you are likely to have just before you make your worst mistake. Remember that the wrong decision feels exactly the same as the right decision, until it doesn't. Remember that misadventure is a diagnosis only made in hindsight. That the pain always comes when and where it's least wanted.

"I wonder if I just get one finger on the other side of the muscle, maybe I'll be able to palpate for the nerve between my fingers," Maggie said.

"Now you're thinking like a surgeon," said Al, already somehow privy to the thoughts of surgeons. "Get in there."

The word sphincter comes from the Greek root *sphingein,* meaning to *bind tight.* As such, the job of the sphincter is to keep things in. That's the job of the sphincter. Reader, you know where this is going, don't you? A sphincter is meant to *hold things in.*

Maggie, with a double-gloved finger, pried at the opening to that door, seeking a better angle on an insignificant piece of rectal minutiae. *Knock knock,* her finger said. *No entry,* said the stalwart sphincter, binding tight with surprisingly rigid contractile force. *Hrmm,* said Maggie, with just a hint of valsalva in her belly. *Knock knock,* her finger said.

A body can hold no secrets, not when you hold a scalpel, but a body can hold surprises. A surprise can be a party, a found treasure, a delight, a new day. But a surprise can also be something different. A sneaky finger. A mail bomb. By definition, a surprise is something you are not ready for. As Maggie felt the muscle give way to allow entry, she felt just the slightest moment of pause, a catch in her breath, a sudden regret, like what a bridge-jumper who survived might report feeling on the moment of first fall, when it is already too late.

Finally, after weeks of quiet anticipation, the gaseous distention of Frank T. Blood's rotting belly had found an exit strategy, and Maggie's finger its unwitting accomplice. The muscle body had until now been an inert red rock in a sea of rolling fat, but upon entry it revealed itself to be an active volcano. In a moment, the smell-magma burst forth to become smell-lava exploding into the surrounding sky. Maggie and Al, the unfortunate Pompeiians whose faces had been positioned directly over the mouth of this intestinal Vesuvius, found themselves overcome by a sudden wind that carried with it a concentrated version of every bad thing they had been inhaling for the previous two weeks, with particles somehow small enough to escape through the microscopic holes of their respirator masks, but large enough to overpower the admixture of menthol, lavender, and cedar that had been holding down the olfactory fort. A barely audible sound accompanied the release, not flatulence exactly, more like a quiet, insistent siren that only Maggie and Alice could hear. *WEE-ooo-WEEeeee-OOoooooo-weeeeee,* it said, right into their bare ears, as Frank T. Blood's bloated belly deflated and his two iliac crests rested firmly back upon the table in relief.

Maggie and Al's eyes met in pure panic, as Maggie instinctively pulled her finger off the sphincter-trigger and hid it behind her back. A millisecond later the smell hit, and they were overcome with a horror-nausea that pulled their stomach contents up and into their mouths before they could stop them, perhaps to provide some alternative sensation to the smell at hand, as if their bodies were saying *look, it's not great, but it's all we got and it's better than whatever that other thing is.* Suddenly the masks were off, their bare faces exposed to the elements and looking for somewhere to deposit their vomit.

The vessel that had presented itself first was a bucket under the table, a bucket the group had referred to as "The Bucket" (because that's what it was, and the limits of their creative nomenclature had been reached when they had named Frank T. Blood). This bucket was the repository for all of the parts of Frank that had been removed during the course of dissection — triangular sheets of skin, globules of fat, partial lengths of superficial muscle that had been removed to reveal the deeper ones beneath; these were piled up in the bucket to be kept with Frank's body when he would eventually be cremated. This was not an ideal place to escape the smell, being full of smell itself, but in the moment it was the best they could do, the only other option being to splay their vomit on the floor for all to see. Even in this crisis, Maggie felt her midwestern decorum pulling against that option.

So it was that Maggie and Al found themselves heaving breakfast burrito and soy latte and gatorade and hydrochloric acid into a pool of discarded human flesh, each heave prompting a cycle of disgust that called up another heave, over and over and over and over again. Maggie's eyes and nose watered in the act, adding her tears and her mucus to the vile bucket soup (or stew, perhaps, given the proportion of solids to liquids).

"I," Al said as a partially-digested Adderall projected from her mouth, "might not be," followed by a fountain of bile, "an ass man anymore."

"Don't," Maggie said, her birth control pill landing with a *sploosh* as it shot from her body forcefully in a tsunami of green tea, "make me laugh."

This continued on, Maggie puking and laughing and groaning, Al yakking and joking, the two in their own world of humor and misery as the world revolved around them in the midst of this airborne toxic event.

"Hey," Jess had said, raising her hand, and backing away toward the door, "*Hey*, Doctor Bald Man." She had inadvertently used their joke name for the man in her panic, a moment she would replay in her mind with regret for at least a decade. "We need help back here."

As the penumbra of smell expanded into the room, nearby students raised their heads from their own anal triangles, grimacing and putting down their scalpels before clearing out from the blast zone. Maggie and Al remained tied to the bucket by powerful emetic forces, but everyone else took haste toward the door and fresher air.

"HEY," Jess repeated more loudly as she joined the wave of retreat, "SOMEone needs to HELP THEM."

Through this ocean of pain, as if through a parting Red Sea, Dr. Bald Man came into view.

It was his time.

He charged like a line captain into battle, pulling an extra mask over his face, calling with him the ranks of tired and hungry surgical residents who reluctantly marched behind like obedient infantrymen.

"Bring your scalpels, folks," he said, with a tired conviction that suggested he'd seen this before. "It's time for emergency surgery."

Maggie and Al hadn't so much left the lab that day as they'd been ejected from it, once the surgical residents had made it clear their retching presence was no longer welcome. Maggie wasn't sure how she'd made it out. She had a sense memory of Al taking her by the hand, of being pulled through a door. She remembered stairs. She remembered the welcome feeling of outside air on her weeping eyes. She remembered a sudden blanket of trees on all sides, as if Alice had pulled her through a portal and into the main plot line of Hansel and Gretl. The brush was thick enough that the hospital building wasn't in view at all, though she could feel its presence. Maggie sat with her back against a tree, as Alice stood a few feet away. They each, somehow, had acquired a cigarette.

Maggie didn't recall lighting it, but she certainly was holding it, and it was lit. She lifted it curiously to her mouth, knowing that's where it belonged, but couldn't bring herself to inhale. Al, in contrast, was puffing hers deeply, rhythmically, the way a person on a ventilator might smoke. Between faux-drags, Maggie draped her cigarette delicately between two fingers and rested her hand upon her knee, allowing smoke to drift up in front of her face in a hazy screen that put everything into softer focus. The smoke made her feel glamorous, like a 1950s Hollywood movie star. A long finger of ash grew precariously at the end of the cigarette as she pondered her new career in film, ash that eventually fell onto the crisp early-fall leaves on the ground below her.

Without speaking, Al came over to stomp her foot onto the now-smoking leaves, and produced from somewhere a coffee can to place on the ground at Maggie's feet. She sat next to Maggie, coffee can between them, and demonstrated how to deposit the ash into it, and Maggie took the hint.

"Should we look on the bright side?" said Al.

"Absolutely not," Maggie responded. "No chance."

"Huh."

Maggie moved the cigarette to her lips and gingerly pulled a little smoke into her mouth, rolling it around her tongue for a moment before puffing it back out.

"I think the surgical residents might have finally noticed us," Al said.

"Yeah, they noticed us alright."

Al shrugged. "All publicity is good publicity."

"I think one of them literally kicked me with their foot."

Al shrugged again. "I think that's a high compliment from a surgical resident."

A post-call surgical resident, at baseline, has a capacity for shit-giving that is rapidly approaching zero. The previous night, that capacity had crested sometime around 2 AM during the third gall-bladder removal of the night, when a bile leak (though unfortunate) had squeezed out the last microliters of adrenaline and prompted a brief second wind, from which it was all downhill. Given this, at 9:00 AM in a dissection lab, when a necrotic gas-bomb had gone off and charged them with performing a highly rare Emergent Posthumous Total Colectomy and Small Bowel Resection, all they had to offer was a kind of brute and instinctive autopilot.

Frank had first been turned face-up, relieving the pressure on his distended colon and stopping the outflow of gas from the anal triangle for just a moment. An incision had been made from xiphoid to pubis, the cut usually reserved for trauma cases and ruptured aortic aneurysms. Instead of a fountain of blood pouring out of this incision, it was a fountain of expanding colon and small bowel that had finally found an escape route, and the residents had laughed later about how it was like one of those prank cans of nuts that springs a snake. The vessels which held the bowel to the aorta had been detached swiftly, and the chief resident had noted with interest a fibrous clot in the superior mesenteric artery that must have prevented the formaldehyde from reaching the intestines during the preservation procedure, a blockage that explained the progressive rot of this intestine that should have been frozen in time. This stretch of gut had most likely been going without blood even before the man's death; he had been rotting in life before he even got here, and had continued rotting on the table until today because of this stubborn clog in his pipes.

Operating on a dead man, it turns out, had been a surprisingly freeing experience. Released from the shackles of blood loss and post-operative healing, the surgeons could work with the speed and flow of concert pianists playing *The Flight of the Bumblebee*, both maximally frantic and completely relaxed. With a sense of smell compromised by months of all-day inhalation of cautery smoke, the smell hadn't bothered them the way it had bothered the two vomiting MS1's who were positioned at the right side of the table and who were barely noticed, until a better angle on the splenic flexure was needed, and the chief resident had tapped them each semi-firmly on the back with a foot as if they were stray cats being told to *move along now,* and Al and Maggie had scurried outside to the woods to smoke cigarettes and forget.

That was how Frank T. Blood, to the relief of everyone, had found himself finally rid of the internal pestilence that had haunted him for weeks before his death of ischemic bowel and sepsis, conditions which had taken away his appetite and replaced it with pain he was too proud to seek care for, and that he had drowned in increasing allotments of hard alcohol until the very end.

Once it was freed, the residents had dumped the entire tube, from sphincter to sphincter, into a double-thick and alarm-red plastic bag which was tied and sealed and labeled and shuffled away into a back room freezer, taking the locus of Smell with it. Some weeks later, an incinerator would receive the contents of this bag, along with the bucket full of Frank-scraps that was mixed with bile and tears, and a separate container full of Frank T. Blood's everything else. The incinerator would forge these odd bag-fellows together in a hot, carbonizing fire. Some of the finest particles, being lighter than air, would rise out of a thick smokestack and into the lower atmosphere, drifting along with the jet stream until they seeded a cloud that might eventually become an early winter rain. Other more macroscopic particles would settle earthward into a small metal box to be sent to Frank T. Blood's nearest relative, a niece who would put it in the trunk of her car to be forgotten for years, until on a whim the ashes would be scattered at the Grand Canyon on a road trip, not because *that's what Uncle Frank would have wanted,* but because the scattering ashes and a southwestern sunset and the desert ochres made for a neat social media story. From dust to dust, but with a number of steps in between.

Maggie's cigarette had burned down almost to the filter, and she dropped the remainder into the coffee can. Alice held out another for her. "Here, maybe you could inhale this one."

Maggie blushed and took the offering. "You must think I'm such an impostor," she said, kind of about the cigarette, but also kind of not. "I feel like I don't belong here at all."

"Of course you don't," Al said. "None of us do."

Al held her own lit cigarette out to Maggie's, touching its tip to her tip for a moment and coaching Maggie to inhale at the same time. She took a gingerly pull that didn't catch.

"Bigger," Alice said. "Like you mean it." Maggie tried again, pulling in a deep breath as she had seen done outside a bar or in the basement of a house party or behind the bleachers in school. "There you go! You're getting the hang of it." As this bit of praise was coming out, Maggie's lungs finally registered the smoke, and Maggie found herself coughing and sputtering as Al laughed. Moments later, as the nicotine wound its way to her virginal nicotine receptors, the coughing and sputtering was paved over with a pleasant sensation of wellbeing and contentedness that took her by surprise.

"Wow," she said, her pupils dilating just enough to saturate the colors in the surrounding trees. "Wow!"

"Not bad, right?" Al looked on like a proud parent.

"Not bad at all. This is just what I needed, Al. Thank you." (She gave this thanks, thinking erroneously that she would look back at this day as The One Day She Ever Smoked). Maggie closed her eyes for a moment, the memory of The Bucket and The Smell and Frank T. Blood fading into the distance. She opened them to find Al holding a flask out to her.

"Here, this'll sweeten the deal."

"Al! Where did you —"

"We deserve it, don't you think?"

Maggie didn't think, in that moment, to ask why Al happened to have this flask of hard alcohol tucked into her pocket. In the moment, it just seemed to make sense that she did have it, being a person who seemed to have everything that was required. The hospital and the bucket and the nausea were a distant memory as she tipped back the flask and drank. *Tequila.* Somehow this dual tobacco-and-alcohol assault on her mucous membranes, still raw from bile and hydrochloric acid, rather than increasing her pain, had burned it away, like a kind of cautery.

"Wooooow," Maggie said, as each inhalation of nicotine built upon the successes of the one that had come before. "Wooow." *Medical Student, heal thyself.*

The two were silent after that, passing the flask back and forth, Maggie coughing less and less as time went on. Maggie felt just the slightest magnetic pull as her hand touched Al's with each passing of the flask; that, along with the nicotine thrill and the sleepy buzz she would normally get with day-drinking had her in a kind of restful, focused bliss she imagined must be the way people feel right before they swear, *no really I drive better this way.*

Maggie finished a third cigarette, dropping it into the coffee can and glancing at her watch. "Shit!" she puffed out with her last breath of smoke. "Class is over. I gotta find Jess to get a ride home." She wobbled a little as she stood, putting a hand on a nearby tree for balance. "Oh gosh, I'm a little drunk." She smoothed her scrub shirt and brushed the pine needles off the butt of her scrub pants, trying to look respectable. "What a surprising day, huh?"

Maggie looked down at Al, who was still sitting on the ground, alternating pulls from her cigarette and her flask, making no moves to stand up.

"Walk me back?" Maggie's voice had that little lilt in it that a woman might use when she was testing the waters of flirtation. Maggie hadn't exactly intended for this to be the tone she took, but she wasn't sorry when it came out that way. Al hadn't explicitly said to Maggie that she was gay, though it seemed to be plainly obvious. Maggie was pretty clearly straight, in every sense of the word, and wasn't really even sure to what end she was making this half-hearted advance, except out of habit. Would her mother be proud or horrified? Maggie was unsure. Here she was, though, speaking with her vowels a little elongated, the end of her sentence drawn up into a question, her head tilting to one side. She was leaning back against a tree now, hands on her hip bones in a way that she had seen other women do to emphasize their waist, her tousled hair falling out of her ponytail and in front of her face in a way she hoped was charming in its mess.

Al looked at Maggie, looked at her own flask, and then looked back, eyes casting up and down in saccades between Maggie's shoes and her eyes. She sighed and pulled her mouth to one side. "You should know I don't shit where I eat."

Maggie sobered up a little as the half-smile came off her face and she stood up straighter. "I wasn't. . .asking you to shit anywhere. For the record."

Was she? Probably not. Surely not.

"Of course not. But you know, I just thought you should know."

Maggie nodded quietly, taking her hands off her hips and crossing them in front of her chest like armor. "Yeah, good policy. *Great* policy." Her lips pursed together and her eyebrows furrowed in agreement. "Excellent policy, Dr. Power. Very. . .*professional.*"

"Believe me, it's not that I don't —" Alice's eyes were sending a message that Maggie couldn't parse. "I just. . ."

"Yep, like I said. Great policy."

"Maggie, you *know* you're not — not *really.* You know."

"You don't have to explain, Al. You really don't! You put your shit wherever you want. I gotta catch Jess before she leaves without me. She probably doesn't have any idea where I am. I gotta run."

Alice looked at her with a face that Maggie would see in her daydreams for weeks later, a face that would act as a kind of Rorschach test. Was it pleading for her to leave or pleading for her to stay? Either way, she took Al at her word, turned on her heels, and steadied herself for a moment before walking back to the hospital.

"See you tomorrow?" Al said, as Maggie walked away. Maggie didn't respond, and just kept walking.

This is the system that produces a doctor. The system may be a high-gravity exoplanet that is not fit for human habitation, but this is the system that produces a doctor, and you want to be a doctor, don't you? So you put on this nicotine spacesuit and you keep going. The system is producing the desired outcome.

CHAPTER 5

PGY10

Having survived to the end of orientation day, Maggie stood waiting for the tram, fulfilling the promise she'd made to Joan not to avoid it. One hand tapped its fingers on her thigh, left right left left, right left right right. The other hand reached into her messenger bag to give her cigarette box a squeeze to confirm its continued presence.

Al ain't dead, called a voice from the cigarette box, *she's just hidin'.* It was Frank's voice, again. Maggie didn't question its provenance or its reality or its intentions. She squeezed the box again. *She ain't dead,* the voice said again, *just hidin'.*

Hidin' where, Frank? Maggie tried to communicate with the voice or specter or thought or hallucination or whatever Frank was in that moment. *Hidin' WHERE?*

To that, Frank had no answer, and Maggie was left gazing out over the city, as a vivid sun shone over the horizon and reflected sun beams off the river and through a thin haze of smoke that had settled along the shore, evidence of ongoing combustive activity across the city. Behind her, two nurses traded dumb-intern stories while pitching each other their respective side hustles selling jewelry or hand lotion or body wraps. *If I make it to platinum level, I'll be earning enough to quit my job,* one was saying to the other. *Oh god, that's the dream, isn't it.*

There isn't a single person working in health care who doesn't have an exit strategy, or wish they did. Not one, Maggie thought.

Maggie waited while the tram car made it to the top, watching as the thick cables spun over their visible gear shafts, a little too fast for her liking. The cable was thick for a cable, but relatively thin (Maggie thought) to be supporting the full weight of the fifty human beings who were about to depend on it not to plummet them two hundred feet down onto the hillside. *Forget about the cars, how often do they inspect the cables?* Maggie thought as the doors opened, and before she could answer it, she was in the car, suspended on those cables, not looking down but imagining the view anyhow. She dug into her phone for distraction, flipping through true crime and missing person podcasts, thinking she might get some ideas on the way down. Her stomach dropped as the tram doors closed and the descent began.

What do you think, Frank? Which one sounds good? She knew Frank wasn't really there, of course. Obviously, she knew. Of course. But that didn't mean he couldn't help.

Wonder what burned last night, Frank said, *n' who burned it? Seems to me there's been a little too much smoke round here for our own good.* Maggie looked down and saw her thumb was poised over a podcast called *Burn Report*, which promised to *Uncover the Real Identity of The Famous Burning Man.* The thumbnail had an image of a local bridge with flames imposed onto the suspension cables, and a shadowy figure in the foreground.

Excellent choice, Frank. Very timely. Maggie popped her ear buds in and pressed play.

This week on Burn Report, a middle-aged woman's voice came on, *we talk to someone who claims to have come face to face with the man himself.* There was a smash cut sound effect, and a younger person's voice came on in an opening teaser. *I saw this dude. I saw him. He was seen by me.* A low vibrato of bass was rising underneath the dialogue, and the tiny ossicles of Maggie's ears clattered together as the tram picked up speed. *But was the person they saw the Burning Man, or was it all just . . . smoke and mirrors? Today, we chase our hottest lead yet to a dumpster full of bubble wrap deep on the east side of the city.*

While she listened, Maggie imagined herself zooming out at a distance above the dangling glass capsule, observing it like a passing cloud. Joan had suggested this technique for Maggie's fear of flying, and it seemed applicable here. Against the advice of the same therapist, Maggie's cloud-visualizations almost always ended with an oversized eagle (or sometimes pterodactyl or dragon when she was feeling whimsical) plucking her plane right out of the sky, looping wildly over the landscape before dropping her directly into the ocean and drowning her and all the other occupants. Somehow, to Maggie, the near-certainty in her mind that she would die on each trip was its own type of comfort, and the idea of doing it in the mouth of a majestic bird or an extinct reptilian demi-god offered a glory that gave her dumb life some meaning. That way when she zoomed back in, broken from her self-induced trance, she would actually feel disappointed that such a grand end had not come to pass, and that she was just safely being transported from point A to point B in a mundane human mechanical invention. As she was today.

Our guest today goes by the online handle, @flaminhot451, and they moderate the most popular subreddit in the city, r/therealburningman. Welcome, welcome. How would you like me to address you?

Doe, if you don't mind.

Doe, tell me about tracking an entity that is famously unpredictable. What do you have that the Arson Unit investigators don't have?

Belief, that's what.

For most of human existence, our kind have been flightless, lumbering bipeds with poor night vision and dumb close-together eyes that mostly focused on the world right in front of our noses. And yet, here Maggie was, staring down at lines of tiny toy cars marching like ants down the highway, hearing the disembodied voices of two distant people whose conversation was now long over, her body hovering over the trees and houses.

Everything has a pattern, the young person was saying, *even chaos has mathematical laws that must be followed. We were confident that with the right machinery and the right inputs, we could start predicting their next move.*

Just nestled within the landscape below, Maggie spotted a hammock strung up high between two cedar trees, a pop of electric blue fabric just visible under the canopy of forest green. It was at least twenty feet off the ground, a strategy to avoid the endless camp sweeps that the new city administrator had set upon the hillside next to the hospital.

All we needed was all the fire information that came before, and we got probabilities for what would come after.

The car rocked slightly as it reached the bottom, and Maggie was dumped out onto the waterfront amongst the crowd of fast-walkers heading home to no doubt dogs and kids and partners and other entities that held the promise of home and hearth. Maggie, absent any of those, also walked eagerly and with purpose. Her building was just a few blocks away, one of several blocks of nearly identical condo high-rise compounds built with the express purpose of housing hospital workers and the adjacent economies that tended to spring up in their wake.

He may think he's choosing at random, but he's not. None of us are.

As she walked, Maggie reached into her bag to squeeze the cigarette box again, to see if she got anything from it. No response.

I don't want to exactly reveal our methods, Doe was saying, *but suffice to say the tools we used are available to anyone these days.*

Maggie arrived at the alcove next to her building, leaned on the wall and took her mask down under her chin, taking deep breaths of the alleyway air that smelled of refuse and urine and a hint of smoke. Her own smoking habit had turned down the volume on all smells over the years, and made even this foul odor tolerable. Interesting, even.

It only took about five days for one of our predictions to be correct. Five days.

As she lit her cigarette and took the first drag, the intrigue was interrupted by a vibratory buzz in her pocket and a staccato ring in her ear, as if an extremely local fire alarm had gone off as she lit up.

Her eyes popped wide, and for a split second she had the thought it was Al calling her back. She looked down at her wrist.

Christopher, it said.

She looked around the alley, suspicious that somehow her ex-husband had known to call at just that moment, just to interrupt a smoke. She wouldn't put it past him. She pulled the phone out of her pocket and stared blankly through three vibratory cycles before giving in and answering.

"Hey." Maggie tried to sound friendly, not rude, but also a little busy.

"Hey."

There was a pause as Maggie let the silence hang like a beaded curtain between them. She muted the microphone in order to take in a drag. Chris, always a detective when it came to these kinds of things, was not fooled.

"Maggie, are you smoking again?" It was a kind tone, not accusatory, like the tone your therapist might take with you. Like you can tell me your secrets and we will work through them together and without judgment. Chris was a master at this.

"None of your business, but no, I'm not." No matter the tone, this line of questioning always brought out the petulant teenager in Maggie.

"Glad to hear it, then." Chris had learned not to push too hard on this button, as Maggie's nicotine receptors had a tendency to defend their territory mercilessly. Maggie took another drag directly into the microphone for comedic effect.

"Did you just call to bust my balls?" Was that Maggie's voice, or Frank's, working through her? She honestly wasn't sure.

"Jeez, Maggie, what's gotten into you?"

Christopher could have been here with her. He had been offered the job, the signing bonus, the waterfront condo, the loan repayment, all of it. As much as Maggie had chosen to leave, Christopher had chosen to stay behind. He hadn't been working in the hospital on the day of the incident, but it wouldn't have mattered. Christopher would have chosen to wallow in the emotional wreckage that had followed, because it was his nature. The only comforts he required were the comforts of decay; the swamp of broken cabinets, unscrubbed floors, supply chain disasters, and piles of paper faxes. His home was and always would be too-small double-occupancy rooms packed with four patients, too-thick computer screens affixed to the wall with broken accordion-arms that were always either stuck at their zenith or drifting aimlessly to the floor, doors that were hung 10 degrees off plumb; these were as good as cash to a man like him. His own suffering was not an unfortunate byproduct, but rather, it was *the point,* and he truly didn't understand why others couldn't or wouldn't live off of this same fuel. The system was Michaelangelo, and he was its David, somehow more beautiful for being broken, the system's most glorious and enduring achievement.

Maggie had wanted to belong there, but she just didn't. Now here she was, and there he stayed. Did she belong here? Did she belong anywhere?

"I'm sorry, Maggie. I don't mean to give you a hard time. I just worry about you."

Maggie was gazing from her alley shadows across the waterfront and out onto the vast, sparkling water that constrained the city, dotted boat wakes dashing across the surface heading someplace, setting sun splashing long shadows onto the concrete. Her mind caught on the jagged edge of the news of the day, and she gasped.

"Oh my god, I have to tell you something."

"Oh? Really?" Chris's tone was hopeful, and Maggie wrinkled her nose in regret.

"Um, it's not pleasant. It's something I found out today. I ran into Jess and Marcus in the lounge."

"Oh, are they okay?"

"Yeah, yeah, they're fine. It's um, hm. It feels weird to say it, actually. Alice. From med school? You remember Al Power?"

Pause.

"Yeah, Maggie. I remember Al. Of course you know I would remember Al. *Obviously* I would remember her. Is she still an asshole?"

There were few people that would get this reception from Christopher, but Al had been under his skin from day one.

"Well, um, *no*, actually. She's not."

"Ha! How's that possible?"

"Well, she's dead, for one."

Al ain't dead, a voice said in her ear.

Not now, she said back to it.

Another longer pause. Maggie heard a long sigh on the other end, and had a picture of exactly the way Christopher's thick eyebrows were probably furrowed in concern, one hand running through his thick, curly mop of hair in thought.

"Shit."

"Yeah, shit. She, um, well. At least people are saying she's dead. *Supposedly* dead."

There, are you happy?

"How is that so?"

"Jess and Marcus told me that — they said she maybe, well, she. . .lost her license, and then. . . you know."

Maggie didn't need to say anymore. A doctor understands the inevitability of the story. A doctor is a person who understands their profession to have the highest rate of certain things in this country, a person who statistically has lost at least one colleague to that thing, a person who has given up the freedom of their youth for the promise of autonomy and respect that never will arrive, a person who toils in a dark tunnel towards a promised light that often turns out to be a dumpster fire. A person who meets certain checklist criteria for conditions they can't seek treatment for without significant professional catastrophe. A doctor knows what comes next. One doesn't need to speak it.

"Are you okay?"

For some reason, that earnest expression of care was what finally broke Maggie's eggshell, and her eyes again moistened with tears, (*twice today,* was either a thought or a voice she heard, *get ahold of yourself Owens*) and her throat became tight and threatened to crack as she replied.

"Um. I don't know, actually."

Chris had a way of extracting emotional truth from her, an ability she had once thought was good for her.

Get ahold of yourself, Owens. There's work to do. It was Frank T. Blood's voice, after all. Insistent, disruptive. Maggie clenched and unclenched her fists. *Get. Ahold. Of. Yourself.* Maggie took out an earbud and cleaned out her ear with her finger, as if the voice were coming from some bit of wax stuck within it.

"I could visit? I've got a golden weekend coming up." Christopher, on the other hand, was soft, pleading. Maggie didn't say no out loud, stifled by what she didn't know. Instead, she just sighed loudly into the phone, took another drag, and then held the silence.

"Yeah, I guess that wouldn't be a good idea, huh? I just want you to be okay. I'm sorry about Alice. I know how much you liked her."

"Well, I know you hated her. I don't know why I even told you."

"Ouch, Maggie. Would it be okay if I called back tomorrow when you've had time to process?" Maggie agreed, offering a meek apology before she hung up the phone. Christopher had done nothing wrong after all, which was exactly the problem.

She took one last drink of the view, crushed the last bit of flame from her cigarette against the brick wall, and tossed the butt down a sewer grate. She wiped her tears as she exited the alley and redeployed her emotional armor.

Get yourself together, Owens. There's work to do. Frank had nothing if not direction.

Around the corner, she walked through the mirrored looking-glass doors to her condo building. The building was moderately tall, twenty-one stories of glass and blonde brick whose image would reflect onto the water's surface on a clear sunny day. A sign near the entrance said *Ella, #LiveintheMoment*, a slogan which was supposed to evoke the spontaneity and possibility of waterfront living, but to Maggie and the hundreds of other hospital employees that lived there it mostly evoked a certain emergency birth control pill that shared its name. Down the street were the buildings Daniel, Olivia, Dylan, and Matisse, and Maggie (lonely, perhaps) had started imagining these condo buildings as tall and stoic Gen Z influencer roommates who had complex and messy relationships that were constantly breaking and reforming. At the moment, Ella was crushing on Daniel, who was still in love with his ex-girlfriend Olivia, who had just come out as bi and was herself pining hopelessly after Ella, like a modern-day real-estate *No Exit* in which the tagline had been recast, *hell is other buildings.*

Poor Olivia, Maggie thought as she cruised past the doorman, past the always-crowded elevator and up another windowless staircase to the third floor; a floor that perfectly split the difference between her hatred of elevators, her distrust of ground-floor windows, and her resentment of forced exercise. As she approached, a fob key in her pocket sent a signal that automatically unlocked the door for her. *Honey, I'm home,* she thought, or said; she wasn't sure. She heard the lock whirr and click and pushed inside.

The sight that greeted her as she opened the door had not changed in the weeks since she moved in. A wall of moving boxes, so meticulously packed at first, then hastily packed in the end, sat still piled on one end of the living room, creating a crude cardboard facsimile of the exposed brick walls in the artist's lofts of her youth. Every day in the morning she would contemplate the wall for a moment, consider the probable contents of the boxes, and then leave the task for a future Maggie to manage, a future Maggie who would have need for such things as: a full complement of wooden serving utensils, haphazardly organized photo albums, multiple sizes of Instant Pot, floppy disks full of undergraduate papers. The boxes were stacked upon a base of 15-year-old medical school textbooks whose value as an insulating material likely outweighed their value in knowledge at this point, given the realities of changing medical technology in the last decade and the increasingly inhospitable climate on the other side of the wall.

What a dump, said Frank, quoting Martha in *Who's Afraid of Virginia Woolf,* who herself was quoting Bette Davis. *What. A. Dump!* It was the kind of reference that a man of Frank T. Blood's generation would make.

Yeah, yeah, thought Maggie. *So what?*

Maggie thought she should probably eat. She had neither hunger nor a plan, but understood her probable physical requirement for electrolytes. She opened the fridge, knowing full well it was basically empty, but she couldn't bear to do another night of Postmates. She settled on bread, peanut butter, and 4 pickles, since these were the available options.

"Alexa, remind me to buy some Soylent," she spoke to an Alexa who was not actually there, because she didn't own one. This was a joke that she, in a different time, would sometimes make for Christopher's benefit, and now made solely for her own. She stood in the kitchen and took down the sandwich efficiently as she contemplated her industrial wall of junk.

Frank, from behind her shoulder, also took stock of the wall, and let out a belly-laugh. *Who the fuck is Alexa,* he said. *And what's she got to do with finding our woman?* It was not clear what was so funny, but the laughter continued. Perhaps Frank was drunk, Maggie thought, like Martha in *Who's Afraid of Virginia Woolf.*

"Alright, alright, alright," said Maggie, out loud. *"Alright."* The laughter stopped.

She sat on the steel framed futon that acted as both her couch and bed (having taken no real furniture from Missouri) and surveyed her sad apartment. The tipping boxes, the sparse furnishings, the trash can full of take-out boxes. The refrigerator, with its shelves empty but consuming power anyhow, creating a tiny winter in the middle of autumn, while simultaneously contributing to some endless, overheated summer in the near future. She thought of Al's apartment, the last time she had seen it, so neatly coiffed and sterile. Was it still that way now? Had it been preserved in amber, like her voicemail?

She opened up her laptop.

Al Power, she typed into Google, not sure exactly what she was looking for. Some evidence? Evidence of what? She would know it when she saw it. Either proof of life, or whatever the opposite of that was.

Did you mean AI Power? Google inquired, assuming that Maggie had transposed an ell for the i in AI. *Showing results for AI Power.* There were a dozen entries for *Smart Home Generators.* A kid's TV show. A Wikipedia entry for a K-pop girl group. A nutraceutical company advertising *"A Breakthrough Nootropic Cheat Code to Unlock Your Focus!"*

Alice had mentioned this problem to Maggie over frozen sections of Frank's brain in the Gross Anatomy lab, as they had delineated his *nucleus accumbens* from his *hypothalamus*. "The problem with Al as a name is that it just looks like AI when it's written. I might just change my name to AI to make it easier on everybody," Al had said. "Seems like it couldn't hurt. Might open up some job opportunities."

"How about All Power," Maggie had suggested. "Something to live up to."

"I like the way you think, Owens," Al had said, as she cut a *carpaccio*-inspired thin slice of thalamus off of Frank's brain, and she laughed the thunderous laugh that made Maggie feel truly accomplished every time she had managed to trigger it.

Even now, knowing what she was typing, Maggie's own brain kept tricking her when she saw the name *Al* written out, the little voice in her head trying to say Ay Eye when her eyes reached it.

That's evidence, Frank said, *everything is evidence in an investigation.*

"Good point, Frank," Maggie said. Given that name and the invincible confidence that came with it, how was it possible that Al had been bested by a dumb medical board? A woman with a name like that lives in the middle of the Venn diagram for people voted Most Likely to Succeed and people voted Most Likely to Commit a War Crime. A person with a name like that doesn't go quietly out of this world with a second-hand SocialEyes message. A woman with a name like that goes out in a blaze of fucking *glory.*

Keep digging, Frank said to her. *You gotta scratch under the fingernails to get to the grit.* Maggie wasn't sure what this meant exactly, but she felt inspired by it anyhow.

"Alice Power, MD" she tried again, this time in quotes, asking more specifically for what she needed, a skill she had been told in therapy to work on in her personal relationships but that she mostly applied in practical settings. This did return a list of results related to doctors named Alice Power, of which there were somehow enough to stretch through multiple result pages. Encouraged, she scrolled through the options.

A neuropsychiatrist in upstate New York. An orthopedist in Texas. A pediatrician in Oklahoma. Internists in south Florida and central Missouri and west Texas. Enough to fill a whole hospital from soup to nuts, but none to paralyze her with their blue eyes or delight her with a crude joke about the *pollicis longus* or to brush their hand against hers maybe-not-on-accident in the Green Team workroom while they toiled at 2 AM on admission notes in third year. None of the pages were tagged with *in memorium* or *obituary* or had headlines like *Scandalized Local Doctor Loses Hard-Fought Battle with Alcohol*.

Not finding her Alice in the fray, she tried narrowing down further. *"Alice Power, MD"* — she paused here for a moment and looked away while she typed —*"obituary."* She looked back at the screen. Here was a 76-year-old funeral director from Maryland whose website hosted a number of obituaries but who personally seemed to still be among the living. Elsewhere a 45-year-old nephrologist from Little Rock who died suddenly of Leukemia and whose family asks for donations to the Livestrong Foundation in lieu of flowers. An 88-year-old emeritus psychiatrist from upstate New York whose claim to fame had been a specialization in Rorschach testing. No 38-year-old west coast surgeons whose lives had spiraled out of control and ended suddenly with only a secondhand SocialEyes post to show for it. Is it possible to die and leave behind no trace? No flowery memorial in the local paper? No official announcement at all? Is SocialEyes what counts as necessary and sufficient these days?

Maggie wasn't one to give up easily though, her online search skills having been forged in the fire of first generation internet dating. She felt confident she could find something, somewhere. In the *comings and goings* section of an alumni newsletter. In the comments section of a hospital's Yelp review section. In an Instagram post of a second cousin somewhere. However, she was growing frustrated. She sighed and clicked exasperatedly around to paywall sites that offered to *Find Anyone for 99.99*, wondering if she should just bite the bullet. But if Al was really dead, that wouldn't help, and if she wasn't— it shouldn't be this hard to confirm it, should it? Or should it?

I've been telling you she ain't dead, Frank said. *I don't know what you think you're going to find in the obituaries. You gotta be lookin' for LIFE.*

Maggie nodded in agreement, pulled out her phone, and without thinking, dialed Al's number again. This time, no rings, just *you know who you reached.* Her eyebrows furrowed and she hung up. She still couldn't bring herself to leave a message.

She wondered if she could search for family members, someone else who could confirm the facts for her. Someone who would have had to go to a morgue to identify an actual body. *Is that still a thing?* And did Al have family willing to do it? Surely at least one person, in that circumstance. A brother, perhaps one who would send a message on SocialEyes. She felt an impulse. She still had Jess' phone number in her contacts; she hoped it hadn't changed.

hey jess, it's maggie. question for you.

Hey Girl! What's Up! On the Peloton 🚴

was there no funeral?

No, I don't think so. Too sad, maybe?

an obituary?

Doubt it.

cold-hearted.

You know Al borrowed a lot of money from people.
A LOT.

like, a fake your death amount of money?

Maggie, you're bumming me out.

just sayin

maybe Al ain't dead.

Bumming. Me. Out.

maybe she's just hidin'

UNSUBSCRIBE!

Maggie dropped it. *Guess I'm on my own,* she thought.

What am I, chopped liver? Frank spat out his drink with laughter. *Get it, chopped liver?* Well, on her own, except for Frank, of course. On her own, except for Frank.

And her laptop, too, she had that. And the internet to which it was attached, and all the human knowledge and thought which that contained, which was no less than the entire recorded volume of all human history and then some. This was an internet where somewhere, on a Wayback Machine, with the right URL in hand, one could find a Live-Journal page anchored by a pixelated thumbnail of early-college Maggie with dyed-red hair, over the cringe tagline "The world doesn't even deserve me at my best," with Lisa Loeb's *Stay* playing in the background. This was an internet that contained high school yearbook photos embarrassing enough to cancel a Bachelor contestant or liberal comic or gubernatorial candidate. An internet where a dedicated teenage sleuth could ruin the career of a high level sports executive just by connecting anonymous Tweets. Where a savvy 12-year-old could buy cocaine from Romania. So it was just her, and Frank, and her laptop, and the omniscient internet-god, looking for a record of the untimely death of a recently delicensed physician in a major city in the United States. It shouldn't be so hard, should it?

"Whaddya think, Frank. What would you do?" Maggie wondered aloud.

Not believe the official story, that's what. NEVER believe the official story. Even if that's the story you're paid to believe.

What are the other options, then? Maggie started to list them in her mind.

1) The SocialEyes message was sent in error. Perhaps the message was nothing more than an errant communique sent about some other Alice Power to the wrong class president following a wayward Linked-In search by a distraught and distracted family member? Perhaps.

2) The message was sent by Al herself. Maybe Al is still alive and well and practicing quietly somewhere in upstate New York. Maybe Al is living off of her own life insurance money somewhere south of the border. Maybe Al has joined a time-traveling island cult and was required to fake her own death. Maybe.

3) Elizabeth was lying about the message. Perhaps in cahoots with hospital risk management?

These all seemed unlikely, of course. Very unlikely, even. But unlikely things happen every day. Golf balls enter the hole in one shot, full court basketball shots are made by fans chosen at random, lotteries are won by garbage men. Maybe it was even more unlikely, Maggie thought, that Al could actually be dead. Alice Power, who took nothing seriously and had told jokes through even the most miserable points of medical school, couldn't possibly have chosen such a drab and typical end to her mirthful life. *Unlikely.* Al Power, a legend for her ability to puckishly wriggle free of any consequence, how could she have found herself in such a bind as to leave no options out? *Unlikely.* Al, a woman who managed to lead the pack during her Obstetrics rotation in two categories: Most Babies Caught, and Most Illicit Smoke Breaks. *Unlikely.* How is it possible for such a person not to rise from the ashes of whatever mistake she had made?

Unlikely. Al was a survivor by nature. She would just as soon start a secret new life at an anarchist compound in Acapulco than succumb to such a banal insult as a medical board investigation. Maggie tapped her fine-tip pen on the coffee table as her gears were turning, leaving little tick marks of smooth ink as the pen tip kept up the rhythm of her thoughts. *Medical Board Investigation.* The phrase ran a loop around her brain and back again. *Medical Board Investigation.*

Frank let out a staccato *yeet* in excitement, followed by *NOW you're thinkin' like an investigator.*

Medical Board disciplinary records were publicly available! They could easily be searched to at least verify the supposed loss of Al's license, and maybe some of the details, which would be a start. She searched for the state medical board, and was led to a website with outdated clipart graphics and an only barely-functional UX design, which convinced Maggie of the site's authenticity as a government entity. She scrolled through the options: *File a Complaint* and *Verify a License* were in large font on the sidebar, followed by *Find a Doctor* and *Search for A Disciplined Physician* (a missed opportunity, Maggie thought, to juxtapose these two options as *Find a Good Doctor* and

Find a Bad Doctor, but then again medical boards aren't known for their sense of whimsy).

Search for A Disciplined Physician turned out to be exactly what Maggie was looking for, a public portal into various sordid misdeeds perpetrated by physicians and physician-like entities, laid out for public consumption. Here she hoped to find some trail that would lead to an account of Alice's misfortune. She knew from years of risk management lectures that state medical boards always put physician discipline on display in this way; the details are considered public interest.

So here, if the public were so interested, they could peruse a comprehensive list of disgraced names, laid bare in 10 point all-caps Times New Roman. The list extended to the bottom of a long-scrolling page vertically and continued on an additional 25 linked pages. A grid of shame, hundreds of ill-fated physicians long by hundreds of selfish misadventures wide. Each name, when clicked, opened up a PDF file of a legal document, sometimes two or three. At the top would be written, *Oregon State Medical Board vs. [Insert physician name].* The PDF would be crooked, oddly cut, and out of focus, as if the document had been fed haphazardly by a drunk octopus through a series of dilapidated fax machines and scanners on its way to this website, no doubt subject to laws about document handling that were out of date thirty years ago but hadn't been modernized because it would require some state senators to care enough to pass a law.

In theory, since the names were in alphabetical order, Maggie could have gotten straight to the point, could have clicked through to find Al's name nestled in between *Pollock, Melanie Susan* and *Parkinson, Edward Geoffrey.* But she stalled, clicking aimlessly into the A names to get a sense of what was here, and maybe to avoid for just a little while knowing things she didn't wish to know. Instead, she just chose the names that sounded interesting to her.

For instance: Dr. Mark Allen Aston III, who *did prescribe opioid pain medications in excess of accepted practice standards,* or Dr. Constance Emily Brock, who *did engage in consensual sexual relations with Patient A, in violation of the code of ethical conduct regarding sexual fraternization with patients.* The reports were mostly all written in this cold third-party style, referring to the offending physician initially with their full first, middle, and last name, like famous assassins or serial killers, and then just as *Licensee* or sometimes *Respondent.* A few details were given of the offending behavior, and then some combination of reprimand, educational penance, and monetary penalty were assigned. The reports were written with great restraint — at the hand of some withholding sadist on the medical board who knew much, much, more than they were willing to say, but gave you just enough detail to pique your interest. Such as the case of Dr. Peter Marcus Connaughton, who *did engage in explicit text messaging with Patients A through F, during a time period when he was actively monitoring anesthetized patients in the operating room,* or Dr. Albert Delaney Maxey, who *is found to have left threatening voicemails for a nurse in retaliation for reporting disruptive conduct,* and additionally *is suspected to have adulterated food left in a common area with a bodily fluid.*

There was something soothing about this exercise, seeing this truly despicable behavior from other doctors spelled out so plainly. It put into perspective all the smaller offenses that had accumulated in Maggie's own life. What was a secret tobacco habit when there were others out here huffing from the anesthesia gas machines after hours? What's the big deal if you park in the patient parking lot sometimes on rainy days when there was a doctor out there trading sex for oxycodone? The pharmacist may be incredulous that you could have so mindlessly clicked through the five penicillin allergy warnings on that patient with an anaphylaxis history, but did she know that there were doctors out there who had defecated in a staff refrigerator? That there were doctors out there getting arrested for attempted kidnapping? Doctors losing their license for taking a piss inside a rival colleague's locker? For having thrown an unsheathed scalpel at a radiology tech in the operating room?

On one hand, one might think it hard to imagine how the people in these reports had gotten through the rigor of study and discipline from undergraduate to medical school to residency to practice, a progression that takes so much restraint and decorum and people-pleasing and rule-following, and then ended up in the unbridled *id* of these stories, wrecking their own lives and others in careless disregard. On the other hand, Maggie knew all too well how the sharp edges of the medical system could wear down one's defenses and expose the soft underbelly of one's worst impulses. So if you had just a little bit of impulsiveness to start and a vulnerable ego and a little bit of an alcohol problem. . .

Maggie took a deep breath, and clicked into the *P* section.

There she was - *Power, Alice.*

Maggie's cursor was on it, her finger on the corner of her trackpad ready to click, but she just stared at it. She knew she was going to click on it, but maybe wanted to extend her ignorance for just another few moments.

Pause.

Pause.

Pause.

C'mon, girly, what're you WAITIN' for? Are we investigatin' or are we sticking our thumbs up our butts? At the last statement, Frank let loose a guffaw that shook the futon and Maggie's innards with it. *And you'd certainly know about sticking thumbs in a butt, wouldn't ya! HaHA! HAHAHHAHAHAHAHAHAHAHAHAH —*

Click.

Click.

Maggie resisted the urge to read the information through a gap in her fingers, as she would a horror movie. Her hands were down, and her eyes were open. Squinting just a little, but open. It felt like she was reading a teenage diary.

Al's entry was sparse, uncontested, but evocative. *Licensee was reported as impaired to the medical board by nursing staff, and the report was substantiated. Licensee then failed to fulfill the requirements of substance use disorder treatment, and was noted to have smuggled* [a smudge here on the PDF made this part unreadable] *to provide an adulterated urine sample as part of routine monitoring. Licensee is therefore suspended from medical practice immediately, and is fined $10,000 for board costs.* Just three lines, removing Alice from a profession that she had spent ten years and a half-million dollars to pursue. At the bottom of the document, there was the signature of the chair of the medical board in a tall and pointed script that meant business. Next to that was Al's signature, except instead of signing her own name, she had signed in a comically curly script:

Frank T. Blood, Private Eye

Maggie gasped.

Whatta fuckin' asshole, Frank said. *Tryin' to blame ME for her shit.*

"Yeah," said Maggie. "I guess so."

So what now? This report had been posted 7 months ago, according to the date at the bottom. Seven months ago. Seven months. *Seven.*

Maggie saw Al on the edge of her bed, buttoning her shirt as Maggie laid tangled in bedsheets. *Gotta get to the hospital,* she had said. *I got an early case. Lock the door on your way out, will you?*

That was six months ago, as this already-signed PDF was no doubt slowly making its way through the bureaucratic combine and onto the internet. Why hadn't Al said anything?

I could have helped.

Under license status, Alice Power was still listed as *Suspended.* Not *Revoked,* as some others had been, and — pointedly — not *Deceased.* Not that this was proof of anything, of course. But maybe it was, as

Frank would say, *evidence*. The SocialEyes post announcing Al's death had been dated from three months ago. That left a 3 month gap between the loss of license and the (supposed) lost battle with alcohol. 3 months where Alice could have reached out to someone for help, could have checked herself into rehab, could have reinvented herself as a health-startup-mogul or an online influencer or a trophy wife or anything that didn't require a medical license. 3 months where she could have become a merchant marine or a bouncer at an exotic dance club or a peer review officer for an insurance company or other things that could be performed while drunk or otherwise impaired.

Why didn't she do these things, she wondered. Pride? Nihilism? Or —

Don't believe the official story, said Frank. *Don't believe it for a second.*

Frank need not worry. Maggie was already a step ahead. *Maybe it's not too late.*

She signed into SocialEyes, implementing now the procedure of gazing at it through split fingers, trying to avoid taking in any more of those gymnastics injury videos without consent. She searched and found the account of Elizabeth, the former-class-president who had received the apparent message from Alice's alleged brother (the brother that, somehow, Maggie had never heard of, in the years of her acquaintance). She sent a quick, hopefully not too cheerful but not too morose, message to Elizabeth. *Hoping to connect with Alice's brother, can you forward me the message? I never got to send my condolences to the family.*

With that, she closed the laptop and stared at the wall of her apartment. "Alexa, bring me a glass of wine," she said, laughing at her own joke. None appeared.

Seriously, who the fuck is Alexa, said Frank, *and can she bring me a brewski?*

Maggie closed her eyes and let out a laugh, a full-throated one that she hoped would somehow summon the spirit of Al. It felt good, and for a second, Maggie forgot herself. When she stopped laughing and opened her eyes, the wall of cardboard boxes was staring back at her, humorless. She noted one box-brick in the box-wall was starting to list sideways as its weight caused a slow collapse of the box below it, like a degenerating spine. She pictured the whole operation tumbling down in the middle of the night, waking her and her downstairs neighbor with a yard-sale of all her earthly belongings onto the floor. She rose to lift the too-heavy box off of its downstairs neighbor. She set it down on the floor next to her futon and lifted the lid.

The box was packed full with carefully banded stacks of paper envelopes bearing her name on the outside, each one containing a tri-fold letter inside. Some of the letters were wrapped in fine stationery with a broken wax seal over the flap and Maggie's name in calligraphy on the front. Others were in long security envelopes with block hand-writing and hastily torn-open flaps. There were photos intermingled throughout, along with a few other mementos: dinner receipts, a pressed flower, a movie ticket. The letters, romantic flotsam from the jet stream of her failed relationships, had traveled with her now for almost 20 years. They'd been saved not for sentimental impulse but rather archaeological, the letters like the changing foraminifera that marked the evolution from the Mesozoic to Cenozoic. Some of these letters marked a brief and hot fire that had burned between her and a college teaching assistant so long ago, back when lovers might still write letters, back when she might refer to someone as a lover.

The ex-lover had been a PhD student at Maggie's university, a teaching assistant for Maggie's sophomore-year organic chemistry course. At the time, she'd been considering a career in chemical engi-neering. She had liked the mix of predictability and surprise in chem-istry, that she could use neat block handwriting to write out the formulas with little dots to represent the electrons, that she could move them around in a way they were forced to obey, that she could combine two pedestrian substrates like acetic acid and isopentyl alcohol and end up with a volatile compound that would fill the room with the aroma of bananas. It always made sense, and (to be honest) came reasonably easily to her, which was another part of the appeal. The teaching assistant had returned her first lab journal with a little sticky note on top that said *See me after class, please,* a note that kicked off an hour of pure panic in which Maggie imagined perhaps her work was so bad, so substandard, that he was going to suggest she drop out and pursue creative writing or sociology or some other soft science. Instead, he had reached his hand out to shake hers (firmly, with one hand doing the shaking and the other gripping the backside as a politician does).

"I just had to meet the person who did this work. It's fantastic," he had said as Maggie let out her breath. "You're a natural. Can I take you out for coffee?"

At the time, their dalliance had felt intense, exciting, fated. One day, a few months in, she had been laying *post coitus* in the twin bed of her dorm room, while the TA had trailed a lazy hand up and down her inner thigh, staring up at its apex adoringly.

"Maggie, I think you might have special healing powers, I really do," he had said, directing this more to the vagina than to the woman attached to it.

"Oh, yeah?"

"I'm not joking. Since you've come into my life, I'm sleeping better. I've been running longer. My work is better, too." The TA's hand wandered suddenly further north as he said this, surprising Maggie and causing her to gasp with not exactly pleasure, a sound she had followed up with a little giggling moan anyhow to signal that it was fine, good even, that he had surprised her in this way.

"I've been thinking you should go to med school," the TA had said, as Maggie squirmed in a way that would have been perceptible to someone who was trying to perceive it. "I think you should be a doctor."

"Med school? I dunno, I was thinking I'd get my PhD. I'm signed up for Polymer Chemistry next semester. Professor Schofield thinks I'll be good at it."

The TA had groaned, and then laughed a bit. "Polymer Chemistry is just such a sausage fest, Maggie, I think you'll hate it." He had gripped her thigh in a way that was legitimately painful as he said this. *Ow,* Maggie had thought, while giving another encouraging little moan in response. "Besides," he said, "why would you want to waste your special powers in a dumb laboratory with a bunch of poindexters?"

This had been the refrain for the rest of the semester, and Maggie came to believe that perhaps she *did* have some kind of healing gift, a destiny to become a doctor that would be wasted on research or industry, an *obligation* even. So she had changed her planned course load from advanced chemistry to pre-med, and then had just stayed that course even after the TA had moved on to shall-we-say-*greener* pastures six months later. He had eventually become a professor at the university, though he'd recently lost this job (Maggie had heard) in the Mass Extinction Event that was the #metoo movement. It turns out, his office-hours-to-bedroom pipeline had only become more well-traveled once he had his own tenure track. No doubt there were many boxes of old letters spread amongst the sad and lonely condos of divorced women in STEM to prove it.

Maggie chose a letter at random and opened it. *Would but I could live in a world without friction,* it said, *I could traverse your curves in endless circles, forever.* Maggie groaned in agony, thinking of how charmed she was by this once upon a time.

Is this what the kids mean when they talk about Tinder, Frank said, looking down at the box, *because this shit looks like it would start a great fire if you know what I mean.* Frank had a knowing, urgent tone with this, and Maggie puzzled for a second about what he could mean. *What're you waitin' for, little lady. Sun's gone down, you know. Alleyway's empty. Burning Man'll be out soon.*

It took her another beat, but she caught his meaning. She lifted the box and walked to the sliding glass door, threw the latch, and walked out onto the narrow balcony. The balcony faced a brick wall, but if she craned her neck all the way to the right, she could enjoy something the real estate listing had called a "peek-a-boo view of Puget Sound." It had come at a price cut that allowed her to purchase it outright when she had moved, thanks to years of frugal Midwest living, a generous signing bonus, and a worker's compensation settlement she had received after the incident at Jackson County Memorial, along with the recent crash of a housing market that somehow, for the first time, she had timed just right.

A modest rain was starting to fall, and the outer cardboard of the box was getting dotted with thick droplets as she stood in the rain. She hoisted the box onto the narrow railing, where it teetered carelessly in the liminal space between artifact and garbage. She looked below to the alleyway and tracked her eyes to a dumpster not 100 feet to the left. Close enough, she thought.

She let go, deciding to leave the rest to fate. The box stayed put on the railing ledge, frustratingly bound by friction and inertia. She considered giving the box a push, then thought better of it. Instead, she turned back inside, sliding the door shut behind her with a little more gusto than usual. When she looked back, the box was gone. She imagined it having landed with a *sploosh* on the pavement below, its contents fanned out across the alleyway and slowly dissolving in the evening rain. The noise of its landing would almost certainly get buried in the groan of the nearby HVAC motor, further obscured by the chatter of the crows that lined the roof, hopefully unnoticed by the other balcony-dwellers with the peek-a-boo view. She had yet to see anyone in the alley who might care about such a mess. *OK, Burning Man. It's all up to you now.* She wondered if that *Burn Report* podcast host had somehow predicted the arrival of this refuse in this alleyway, and was on route to set up a recording apparatus at this very moment.

Frank laughed and laughed and laughed until his laughter turned into a hacking cough that slowly petered out.

"Go to bed, Frank," Maggie said. "I'll take it from here."

Frank obliged, for the moment, and Maggie sat with the silence for long enough for her own curiosity to get the best of her. She went out to check the aftermath. From the 3rd floor, she couldn't make out the faces on the pictures, the half-ripped and punctuated smiles, the shifting eyes. She hoped they'd somehow be gone in the morning when she went down to smoke her cigarette, wondered if she hadn't quite thought this through (of course she hadn't), wondered if she'd doomed herself to find these letters stuck to light poles and shoe bottoms all over the city. But it was done. Tomorrow, maybe, depending on how things went, she'd send the medical textbooks after them. She muttered another silent prayer in her mind to the Burning Man, the impulse to pray having never been fully eradicated even after the slow dissolution of her religious belief. She held that space for as long as her skeptical brain would allow, then turned back inside.

She hit the lights and laid herself down on the steel-framed futon and took one last shuffle of her *p*Value* deck in the dark. She had matched with Jack, the dancing KnockKnock doctor, and with the weed guy. Which meant, conversely, that everyone else had passed. *Ain't that something.* Hovering on the thin red line between insult and gratitude, she fell asleep fully dressed, with the campfire glow of her proximal iPhone disrupting her REM patterns just enough to hopefully ensure a dreamless night.

CHAPTER 6

MS1

Having left Al in the clearing, Maggie rode the Green Elevators alone down to the Morgue level and back to the women's locker room, her cheeks puffy with the angry edema of repeated vomiting. A couple of women in the elevator were chatting about preferred brands of leggings as she had walked on, and she tried not to clock the look of (disgust? horror? pity?) they gave each other as she passed them by to lean against the back wall. She couldn't be sure, but it seemed one had subtly put a hand in front of her face, gave a knowing look to the other, and pushed the button on the next floor down to make an early exit. Not that she could blame them, since she must be exuding the combined aroma of tobacco, alcohol, and rot, even if she could no longer register it.

Maggie, you idiot, what was *that,* she thought on a loop, *what* was *that,* as the elevator lurched down and reactivated her nausea. She tried to look on the bright side; *at least everyone is probably gone and I won't have to explain my face.* She looked at her watch (a real watch, made with gears and not chips, something that was surprisingly common back in this day), and saw that class had been over for two hours at this point. *Damn.* Jess was not exactly the type to wait around. Maggie tried to steel herself for the high likelihood that she'd need to take the bus home, a prospect that was nauseating even under the best of circumstances, and infinitely worse here with a stomach full of bile and a bloodstream full of alcohol and nicotine. She took a deep breath and exhaled just before the elevator reached its nadir. *Get ahold of yourself, Owens.*

As the doors opened, the air surprised her. The Smell, which had only grown increasingly pungent on this floor for the last week, seemed to have dissolved into something less vile while she was away. Was it the effect of the cigarette smoke softening her senses? Was it the bile in her nose burning away olfactory judgment? Or was it really better? She was grateful for the illusion of its improvement anyhow. It still didn't smell *great,* but the *not great* was sterile and chemical rather than the unsettling rot she had become accustomed to. Had Frank's gaseous release been all that was needed, and had the charcoal-scrubbers in the air-handling system somehow taken up the last of it? Better yet, had Frank T. Blood finally had enough of their exploratory bullshit, hopped upon his Harley Davidson, and rode off into the sunset, taking his Smell along with him? Did he mutter a hoarse *Frank T. Blood don't stay where he ain't wanted* to the shocked room on his way out? She pushed through the double-doors at the end of the hallway, lost in the reverie of this fantasy, humming *Livin' On a Prayer* quietly under her breath as she pictured Frank T. Blood engaging in his last act of outlaw rebellion, popping a wheelie on fat motorcycle tires, his flaps of back skin and transected *longissimus dorsi* flapping in the wind behind him —

"Oh!" She jumped, startled to find a human form on the other side of the doors. "Christopher?"

Christopher was there, sitting cross-legged on the cement floor with *Netter's Atlas of Human Anatomy* opened up in front of him, brown hair worried into curlicue spikes on top of his head as he ran his fingers through it.

"Oh!" Christopher responded in kind. "I was. . .waiting for you. You guys, I mean. Where's Al?"

"You were waiting for us?" Maggie felt her lacrimal glands start to contract involuntarily, and she rubbed her eyes to try to disperse the evidence. "For me and Al?"

"Yeah, I have some Zofran. I thought you might need it. I figured you'd need to come back for your stuff, eventually."

Maggie, overcome by this act of kindness in just the moment she needed it, found herself losing the battle between her decorum and her tear ducts, as fat droplets started to fall down her cheeks, embarrassingly. Her mother would be proud, though, to see her daughter crying in front of a tall man.

"Sorry," she said, sliding her back down the wall to sit next to Christopher on the cement. "My eyes are just burning." She rubbed them again to emphasize her point, then held her tear-moistened hands out to receive the anti-nausea pill as if it were a communion wafer. Maggie unwrapped it and put it under her tongue (*don't chew it, let it dissolve,* Christopher directed her), taking in a deep breath through her acid-cleansed nasal passages and letting it out slowly. Christopher turned his head to look at her, and then got a pained look on his face as he focused on something just above her hairline. "Um, you've got a little . . ."

He grimaced and gingerly reached his thumb and forefinger just to the top of her head, flicking a tiny piece of *something* off her hair and onto the floor beside her. "Huh," he said. He was now looking more concerned as he completed a secondary survey of her in the bright hallway light. "Huh."

"What?" Maggie started to run her fingers through her hair when Christopher stopped her short.

"No, no, don't do that." Christopher's eyes were wide, with a look that suggested the possibility of a scorpion or a time bomb on her head.

"What?" Maggie was now frozen solid.

"I, hm. You might, you might want to hit the showers. It looks like you might. . .need one."

Maggie, suddenly self conscious, looked down at her stained scrubs and laughed nervously. "Yeah, I guess so." She changed the subject reflexively away from her appearance. "Hey, have you seen Jess? She's my ride."

Christopher looked down at the floor for a beat, taking in a deep breath before saying: "I can give you a ride home if you need it."

"Oh, I think Jess —"

Christopher shook his head. "Yeah, she left. I won't tell you what she said, but I'm sure you know what she thought."

"Well, whatever it was, she's wrong."

Christopher had just a hint of a smile on his face. "So, do you need a ride, then? I'm headed over to your side of town anyhow." Maggie could catch a hint of *something* in this offer for a ride. She wasn't born yesterday, but thought *what's the harm,* as she considered the nauseating public-bus alternative.

"Sure, yeah, thanks, that would be great."

Christopher's half-smile made it the rest of the way up. "Soooo, where *is* Alice?"

"Outside. I think she'll be out there for a while. She's got some tequila to keep her company." Maggie noticed Christopher's smile briefly inverted at that.

"I thought I smelled alcohol, but I don't trust my sense of smell right now."

"Give us a break. We had a rough day." Maggie stood up to head into the locker room, giving Christopher a too-friendly pat on the knee on her way up. "Guess I'll clean up? I'll be back in a jiffy. Thanks for waiting."

"No problem, I'll just be studying, anyway." Christopher went back to his book, running his finger along the course of the hip adductor muscles they would be responsible for uncovering the next day, mouthing their names silently to himself. *Gracilis, Adductor Magnus, Adductor brevis*, his lips said, as his finger traced the course of the longest muscle in the human body. *Gracilis,* he repeated with his eyes closed. *Gracilis.*

Maggie left him to this task, and she entered the locker room and was immediately confronted with the full-length mirror she usually took pains to avoid. She was taken aback by the figure in front of her and stopped to take it in. Her reddened face was puffy and swollen around the eyes, her jawline rounded by enlarged and angry lumps. Her fingers pushed on the offending mounds. *Submandibular glands,* she thought, proudly. In the midst of all this excess fluid, her cheeks, owing to the caloric deficit of the last 11 days, were somehow sunken and hollow, and her face had taken on the uncanny character of a malnourished and protein-deficient child from a UNICEF flyer. Her scrubs were stained and haphazardly tied, and her shoes had a splatter of *something* creating an abstract pattern upon them that made her shudder.

And her hair. *Her hair.* What Christopher had noticed with a grimace, and had tried to save her hands from running through, were miniscule just-macroscopic bits of fat, muscle, flesh, and vomitus that were creating a speckled popcorn-ceiling effect atop her head, as the fine back splatter from The Bucket had found a willing canvas in her unconditioned hair, the folds and irregularities of her ponytail providing ample surface area for this gray-green mist. Maggie turned away from the mirror, having seen enough, and headed to the showers.

In the shower (ice cold, chosen for maximal numbing effect), Maggie clenched her eyes and mouth impenetrably, pinching her nose shut to keep her orifices isolated from the morbid baptism-by-flesh that needed to happen as the water ran down her body, carrying away with it all the wasted bits of Frank. These morsels traversed the curves of her body to pass through the loosely grated drain and into the sewer system. There, they were diluted in gray-water that would eventually be carried to a nearby water treatment plant, where the water would be cleansed of its biosolids and returned to this selfsame shower in a morbid life cycle of waste and return.

As a child, Maggie had practiced holding her breath in the bathtub while her mother timed, with her personal record sitting at two minutes and sixteen seconds; today, she counted only to 45 before she was forced to breach the gates and take a desperate breath. She tried not to think about the sensation of something on her tongue that was quickly spit out as the breath went in, *probably nothing, probably nothing* as she went back for another rinse. That cycle went on for fifteen minutes, until Maggie peered down at her feet to see the water running clear, ran her hands through her hair to check for stragglers, and found none.

She heard a voice call out from a crack in the locker-room door: "Hey, uh, you okay in there?" *Oh shit,* she thought, having forgotten that Christopher was waiting for her in the hallway.

"Yeah, yeah, sorry — I'll be out in a second." The snap-to-reality was good for her, as she tossed her tainted scrubs in the industrial garbage can, scuttled to her locker, and dressed quickly and efficiently.

"Hey, feeling better?" Christopher said to her in the hallway with what seemed like genuine interest.

"Yeah, yeah I am," Maggie said as they walked side by side to the Green Elevators that would take them up to daylight.

Years later, Christopher and Maggie, the married couple, would tell a mutating version of The Story of The Ride Home to friends and family, one that would condense the horrifying first half of this day into one statement that *it had been a particularly tough day at school.*

This elision is a habit every doctor picks up during training, because when excited friends and proud family ask them *oh my god how's med school going,* those details are not the type of things they want to hear. The type of thing they want to hear is *I'm learning so much it's like drinking from a firehose* and *I really feel like I'm going to make a difference in this world* and *the human body is so fascinating.* Maybe, in some circles, a doctor might add, *do you want to hear a funny thing a patient said to me* or *can you believe what this patient had placed inside their rectum* or *oh my god I stayed awake for 36 hours straight can you believe it.* Rarely, almost never, do people want to hear things like *I was covered in flesh and vomit today* or *I think I've made a huge mistake but I can't quit because I've already taken out a hundred thousand dollars in student loans.* Since the proud faces and enthusiasm of family and friends are all the good feedback a doctor may have left in this world, they leave out any details that might diminish it. If that's lost, what do they have left to get through?

The rest of The Story of The Ride Home, told far and wide over double dates and Christmas dinners and wedding speeches, would focus on the following commonalities that Maggie and Christopher discovered as she rode shotgun across town in his twenty-year-old Chevy S10: the rusted lived-in character of their respective vehicles;

their joint love of tater tots; similarly religious working-class parents; that they had been dreaming at night about Frank T. Blood. *It was like kismet,* Christopher would say later as part of their wedding vows, *the universe brought us together.* Maggie would conveniently leave out any mention of the significant alcoholic buzz she had carried through this ride, and also that her mind (at the time) had been drifting back to Al-in-the-woods as Christopher-in-the-truck was having an electric experience of destined meetings.

In retrospect, Maggie was happy to share Christopher's belief that it was all *meant to be,* because it seemed better to believe than the alternative, and because Christopher had been an objectively correct partner, being stable and kind and rational and well-liked, and being so sure about everything. Christopher, who had volunteered at the needle exchange and the free clinic through medical school, who had brought Maggie coffee every morning from then on, who had never wavered in his choosing of her. Christopher, who didn't snore, who didn't smoke, who would run three miles every day before the sun came up. Al, by contrast, was brash and brilliant and combative and unattainable and uninterested, and of course it was never going to work, of course it wasn't.

At the end of the ride, in The Story, Christopher would describe watching Maggie walk through the door of her run-down apartment building with the thought, *I'm going to marry that girl someday,* and that would be the end of their delayed meet-cute.

The next scene, one that only Maggie was present for, would be left on the cutting room floor. In this scene, Maggie had waited just inside the foyer for Christopher to drive away, then walked right back out and over to the nearby corner store for her first pack of Camel cigarettes and a six-pack of Miller High Life, both of which were consumed alone on the roof of the building until she had reached a state of sufficient forgetting to fall asleep without the fear of what dreams may come. Loving friends and encouraging family and future and past spouses certainly don't want to hear this part of the story, so it is left out.

The system is a forest fire, and your emotions are the underbrush that must be burned in order for new life to emerge. You will be a doctor, and the system is achieving the outcome it desires. The system is working perfectly.

The weeks passed in a blur of increasingly minute body parts, as the four reveled in stripping Frank's now-less-purulent chassis of all its useful parts. They sang gleeful mnemonic jingles about Frank T. Blood to help them memorize things like the anterior flexor muscles of the forearm or the structures of the posterior leg compartment or the tributaries of the inferior vena cava. The other students, who'd avoided their table before the eradication of the smell, now stopped by on occasion to join the singalongs. There were no further surprises, unless you count Maggie and Christopher's surprise dating announcement, after which Al had raised Frank's hands in the air to signal *touchdown* in support.

By the tenth week, only Frank's face remained unexplored.

Frank's cloth mask had stayed on through all of what had come before, through superficial back and pectoral region and posterior thigh and anal triangle and inguinal region and pelvic viscera and external genitalia; it had even stayed on through anterior and posterior triangles of the neck, although the cloth had inched upward and upward and upward, sometimes giving a teasing glimpse of the angle of his strong jaw or the three days of stubble on his chin. Eventually, the day had to come when the whole glory of it would be revealed. Maggie, Christopher, and Jess had already planned a post-lab champagne lunch to celebrate Face-Off Day, as they had called it, in honor of the Nicolas Cage/John Travolta movie they also were planning to screen at Maggie's apartment after the champagne. It was a Big Event. Al was there that day too, though her attendance had gotten increasingly sparse as the term had gone on.

When Al did come to lab, she was fully on point, as if she hadn't missed a day, spinning the scalpel in her hand like a rock drummer waiting for her solo to come up, producing the names of the structures and their attachments at will, she had one of those brains that seemed limitless. In the lecture hall, she would often slide in late to sit in the row behind Maggie, where she could whisper commentary into Maggie's ear to make her laugh, with the added benefit of annoying the ever-present Christopher in the next seat over. But mostly, *mostly,* Al was just increasingly absent.

Maggie had sent her a picture of The Shroud of Turin the night before Face/Off Day with the message, *hope to see you for the big unveiling,* and Al had sent back a pointing finger emoji, a bullseye, a smiling poop, and wind. When Al had finally arrived, she'd posted up at the foot of the bed, far away from the action, as the other three crowded up around the head. ("Feeling a little nauseous," she had said believably, "hope you don't mind if I stand back.")

It only seemed right that Jess, the future dermatologist, should do the honors of unveiling the face, and so Maggie and Christopher each stood on one side, holding Frank's hands in their own as if to comfort him as he crossed over from the darkness into the light. Maggie noticed a slight vibration to the table, which was coming from a tremor in Al's hands resting on the end of the table.

You okay, Maggie mouthed, and Al nodded, smiling her wide smile at Maggie as she lifted a tremulous hand off the table to wipe a bead of sweat that had formed on her brow. *Must really be sick,* Maggie thought, *good she was able to make it today.* Years later, the remembering of this moment will be less benign, more evidentiary, but at the time Al had seemed resilient, un-phased.

In the moment, the day had felt holy, as if the group were early disciples and Frank T. Blood might be laid upon this table to account for their earthly sins. Jess untied the twine around Frank's neck with newly black-manicured nails under her gloves. One, two, three, she counted, and then whipped the cloth off of Frank's face as a magician might.

There he was, for the first and last time. This was not the face from Maggie's dreams, but then again nothing could be, since the dream-face had shifted shapes over the last two months in a way that encompassed all possible human facial features. It was still, even after all that had transpired, surprising. The skin of Frank's face sagged unnaturally off the bone, having undergone a liquefying process of decay, giving him the look of a wax statue partially melted in the hot sun. His eyes were absent, the eyelids taped shut and sunken into the empty sockets. Somehow, in this bizarre repose, with his body wrecked and flayed and decomposed and indecent, Frank T. Blood was still smiling. Between his lips, the tip of his tongue protruded outward in a static, silly little raspberry.

They all stood in silence for a moment, unsure how to properly react. Al had broken the silence with a song.

"Oohhhhhh, Frank T. Blood, had a house full of gas, Ohhhh Frank T. Blood! Frank T. Blood! Until he got too full and he blew it out his ass, Ohhh Frank T. Blood! Frank T. Blood!" Then she stopped singing, and let out a loud and joyous *BAH! BahAH! BAHAHAHAHA!* She could not contain her glee, and soon it poured out of her and shook the table even more, until Maggie was infected with it and began smiling and then laughing, and then Jess, and finally Christopher in spite of his better judgment joined them in mirth, chuckling quietly under his breath. Marcus, from the table next to theirs, had peered over and said, *well would you look at that,* before joining in, and eventually the whole room, all 84 students, plus the bedraggled surgical residents and Dr. Bald Man himself, all circled by to pay their respects to old Frank T. Blood, that stinky sonofabitch, who it seems had gotten literally the last laugh as he shuffled off the chains of his pestilent body.

The laughter had died down after only a few minutes, and Christopher eventually broke the mood by opening up his dissection guide. They were meant to start by exposing the *orbicularis oris,* a muscle that encircles the lips and mouth, and for this they were forced to push the tongue back into Frank's mouth and out of the way, a maneuver that was surprisingly difficult owing to the edematous turgor that had overtaken Frank's rogue tongue. Maggie and Jess and Christopher had become so focused on the task at hand, that they didn't notice for several minutes that Al wasn't saying much, and when Maggie finally turned to say, "Hey Al, do you want to —"

She was already long gone.

Chapter 7

PGY10

Maggie startled awake at 5:15 AM as an oppressive morning sunbeam cut through her blackout curtains. Her phone was buzzing under her shoulder on the futon. She rolled her eyes behind their lids and pulled it out to answer.

"Christopher, when I said you could call, I didn't mean at the ass crack of dawn," she said with sleepy annoyance. On the other end of the phone, she heard Christopher clear his throat and sigh, but he didn't say anything. "What, you got nothing to say now," Maggie said curtly, and the other line clicked off and she was met with silence. *What a jerk,* Maggie muttered under her breath as she sat up.

Who you callin' a jerk? Frank asked. Frank's voice had made it through the night, and was there to greet her this morning. Maggie swung her feet over the side of the futon and onto the carpet, curling her toes to catch the shag between them.

Rise and Shine, sweetheart. We got work to do, Frank said. Maggie stood and looked around the empty room to confirm its emptiness.

"You stay out here, Frank. I gotta shower," she said loudly to the shadow of her jacket hanging by the door.

Seems unfair, what with how much of MY body YOU'VE seen. Frank laughed at his own joke. *Besides, I ain't got eyes, anyway. They took 'em, remember?*

"Just! Stay out here. Make me some coffee, if you don't mind."

Who do you think I am, Alexa?

"Goddammit Frank, just let me wake up."

Maggie closed the bathroom door and undressed to hop in the shower. As the shower hit and her brain came online, her mouth fell open and a bit of shampoo ran into it, the bitterness on her tongue triggering a cough. She ran out of the shower naked, still half-soaped, and ran to the futon to retrieve her phone again. She ignored a wolf-whistle from Frank as she opened up her recent calls, finding the one that had just woken her.

Incoming Call, it said, *5:14 AM, Al Power. 1 minute.*

Maggie's teeth clenched and her breath stopped as she smashed at the button to return the call. As she did, the home screen was suddenly taken up by the image of Maggie's own naked body as she loomed over the phone, and Maggie stared confusedly at it before realizing that she had inadvertently requested a video call. In a panic, as the phone continued to ring, she searched for an option to hide the video, eventually just covering the entirety of the phone with her wet palm as Frank looked on and laughed. When she lifted her hand, the call was disconnected and her nudity was back offline. When Maggie gathered herself to call again with audio, the phone rang and rang and rang, with neither an answer nor a voicemail. *Strange.* After a minute, Maggie gave up.

Had she seen Al's face for a split second before she'd covered the phone, or had she imagined it? Had Al gotten a split-second call and hang-up from Maggie's boobs? She tried the number again, getting still endless rings. She sat and held her head between her knees, covering her neck. The ground moved beneath her feet, but she ignored it until it stopped. When she sat back up, the shampoo-water had run from her head into her eyes, and she felt her nakedness again, so she went to the shower to rinse off.

As she stepped out of the shower, her nose caught a hint of smoke in the air.

"You smell that, Frank?" she shouted through the closed door.

No, maam. Lost my brain, remember? I ain't smell nothin.' You're gonna have to come check it out yourself.

There was, though, the unmistakable sulfurous smell of fire.

Could it be? She dried off, slipped on a robe, and tiptoed to the sliding door. She slid the door open slowly, silently, like a child avoiding the wrath of a surprised Santa Claus, before stepping outside. There on the ground, three floors down on the wet pavement, stood. . . nothing.

No pile of ash. No yard sale of love letters. No dissatisfied smiles or empty promises or half-burned carbon remnants. No clearing smoke to suggest a mechanism for the disappearance. No Elven footprints traveling away from the scene. Just blank space, like the world after the rapture.

Maggie questioned her memory of the prior night. Had she been dreaming about pushing the box over the edge? Her mind was certainly doing unusual things in the last 24 hours; she had to admit that. She looked at the wall of boxes, noting the gap that was indeed still there, suggesting no dream. She looked back outside and extended her gaze down the entirety of the alleyway. Maybe the wind had taken it? There were some cigarette butts collected in the area of the probable abduction. Perhaps an early chain-smoking garbage man? Perhaps the letters had never existed at all? *Either way, I guess they're gone now.*

Her attention was broken by a scratching and a scuffling outside her door. She stood silently for one moment, trying to make out what the sounds could be. A mouse? A wayward cat? The scratching pattern seemed too deliberate, too human. A manager maybe? Surely not this early. A mistake? A serial killer?

"*Frank!*" she whispered. "*What do I do?*"

Her adrenal glands were firing off a number of untoward possibilities, and her heart rate shot up.

Well, you answer the door, of course! Frank T. Blood don't hide from nothin'!

Frank was speaking too loudly, and Maggie held her finger up to her lips to silence him. She tried stalking over to the door to peek through the peephole without revealing her presence, but in the process accidentally knocked over a box of dishes, which spontaneously unpacked themselves exuberantly onto the floor with a crash. A souvenir daiquiri glass from her bachelorette party rolled across the hardwood in a wide, imperfect circle before settling at the foot of the door.

A young tenor voice came muffled through the heavy door, "*Something something,*" there was a pause, "okay in there?"

It certainly did not sound like the voice of a serial killer, she reasoned. She erected herself, pulled the robe tie firmly taut, picked up the glass as one might a weapon, and cracked the door open. Was she secretly hoping for a serial killer? She could unpack this someday with her therapist, if she lived to tell the tale. She gripped the glass tightly in her hand as her visitor came into focus through the door.

The person was standing in the hallway with a look of surprise. Young, twenty-something, a smooth face fit with too-large glasses and unruly blue hair, and wearing a white button-down shirt with the buttons all-the-way buttoned up, like a Jehovah's Witness might. However, there were no pamphlets in hand entitled *Are you Ready for Heaven?* Instead, there was a cardboard box, slightly damp, with the inscription OWENS 3:16 on the side. She released her grip on the glass.

The box had been labeled by her moving company, and Maggie had gotten a kick out of how they'd put the colon to make it seem like a bible verse. *For Maggie so loved the world,* she thought. Maggie looked from the box up to the face and realized she recognized it.

"Jax?" said Maggie with shocked confusion. "From orientation?"

Jax coughed, as the surprise of Maggie's door-swing seemed to have knocked loose some frog in their throat. After they caught their breath, they spoke. "I, uh, I was just trying to leave you a note. I know it's early, I'm so sorry. . .but then it seemed like you must be awake, based on, you know, the noise."

"Where did you," Maggie stuttered, looking at the box.

"Oh, OH. Yeah, I found this box in the alley. I assume it's yours; the pictures are of you." Maggie recoiled.

"You looked? At the pictures?"

"I didn't mean to! Just to put them back in the box. I — uh, I *live* here, you know. Down the hall? Um, guess we're neighbors? Small world, huh!" They coughed some more, holding their elbow over their mouth like Dracula would a cape.

"Oh boy," said Maggie. "What luck."

Jax's arm dropped back to their side, and Maggie noticed a fine speckling of gray or black that had been deposited on their shirt from the cough.

"How did you know where I live?"

"Ohhh." Jax rebalanced the box to free a hand to adjust the glasses on their face, a move that seemed to take a great effort, and then gestured to the box itself. "Your unit number was on the side?"

"Oh."

Rookie mistake, said Frank, *Can't believe you gave yourself away like that, Owens.*

Maggie suddenly felt the weight of an accusation at hand and tried to reel through possible explanations for why her personal effects had been found in the public right of way. *Some windstorm we had last night, huh? Must have left the window open.* Before she had a chance to share this lunatic dissemblance, Jax gave her an out. "I figured your movers must have dropped it or something."

"Yeah, yeah, must have, geez."

"Seemed like stuff you might" — Jax took a breath — "want back." They paused again, Maggie noticed, and continued to do so frequently. "I live at the end of the hall" — *breath* — "my unit looks out on the alley" — *breath* — "I was just" — *breath, cough, cough* — "I should have just taken it to the office" — *breath, cough* — "I know." The skin around their trachea was retracting with each breath, and they continued to pause awkwardly between words to take in air.

"Do you actually" — *pause, breath* — "want this box of stuff" — *wheeze, wheeze* — "or should I put it back" — *deep breath* — "in the alley?"

As they spoke, Maggie pulled the sides of her mouth down in something that was both a grimace and a frown. "Maybe it was meant to be in the alley," she said. Jax frowned. Maggie backpedaled. "No, no, I'll take it, I'll take it." Maggie received the box in her arms, and Jax watched from the doorway as she walked over to put it back in the empty space along the box-wall that had been left when she took it out last night. "Will you look at that? A perfect fit. Must have been fate."

"Bazinga," Jax said, standing there holding the door open with one foot, hands clasped in front like a bellhop who was awaiting the promise of a tip. Maggie neither invited Jax in nor excused them to leave, and they remained in this standoff for a moment too long before Jax took the hint.

"Well" — *pause, breath* — "I guess I'll be seeing you" — *cough, wheeze* — "around?"

Maggie waved. "Yeah, yeah I guess so."

The door shut behind them as they turned to leave, and a fit of now-uncovered coughing echoed down the hallway in little plosive bursts as they left, Maggie jumping involuntarily with each burst of *rat-a-tat-tat*. Maggie considered going after them to see if they needed medical attention, or at least she thought she should consider it, though she didn't, really. She lifted the lid off the box to check its contents, now soggy and in disarray. *I guess you were meant to stay with me for a little longer*, she said to the box, placing the lid back on and patting it twice with her hand.

What a nice young man, Frank said problematically, *Wonder why he was really in the alley last night.*

"Frank, why do you believe everyone is lying?"

Because they are, sweetheart. Because they are.

Maggie dressed, gathered her messenger bag and climbed onto her Danskos. She walked back to the bathroom to take a quick peek in the mirror, something she didn't usually do, but Jess' comment about her skin had made her self-conscious. The face looking back at her was recognizable enough, though somehow aged from even a week ago. Women in medicine have a narrow window in which they are neither too young to be taken seriously nor too old to be taken seriously, the way women in Hollywood suddenly go from playing the sexy ingenue to playing the senile grandmother over the span of five years. She wondered where she fit now in that continuum, as new streaks of gray were developing just above both temples, along with increasingly unsubtle crow's feet pointing arrows at her eyes. A distinguished look, she thought. Who cares if it's unfuckable, right?

What are you doing, Maggie, she heard her mother's voice now in her ear, the same voice she had heard when Maggie had told her about the divorce, *you don't want to grow old alone, trust me.* But then again, maybe she did? Couldn't there be value in solitude?

Stop stallin' Owens, there's work to do.

"Yeah, Frank. I'm coming."

Maggie gingerly walked out of her door, looking both ways before stepping through as if a city bus might come careening down the hallway to take her out. Seeing none, she set out for the day. As she walked away, she listened for the *whirring* of the front door's self-locking mechanism that would activate when her key fob gained enough distance from it. The door would wait patiently all day for her return, sending out radio frequency pings *ad infinitum*, like an eager puppy. *See mom, someone* is *waiting for me to come home*, she thought.

Maggie was already cutting it close to get to the workroom on time this morning, but as she walked out into the morning, her feet took her away from the hospital, on a whim. She circled two blocks back to the corner where the Daniel building stood. *Live at The Daniel,* a sandwich board read out front, *You Deserve It!* A threat or a promise, or both. This was where Al had lived, *or could still live,* Maggie thought, standing a few yards askance of the front door and lighting a cigarette. A passerby coughed pointedly at her as they walked through the aura of her second-hand smoke, and Frank yelled behind them to *keep walkin' buddy, it's a free country.*

Maggie couldn't remember which floor Al lived on; it wasn't the top floor, but it had been up there, with a balcony that faced the street. She scanned the grid of balconies for signs of anything identifiable. Had Al owned a red bicycle? A beach towel with Hang Ten written on one end? A collection of hanging potted plants? A pair of skis? Maggie realized at this moment that she knew very little of Al's hobbies. As far back as she could remember, rearranging the major organs of other people was Al's primary pastime.

Maggie picked out a particularly blank balcony five floors up, her eyes drawn there by its contrast to the others. Imagining what the view from the balcony might look like, she grew more sure of it. *That's it,* she thought, *that's the one.* A young woman carrying two large bags was headed now for the front door, and Maggie saw her opening. She squashed the cigarette just as the woman started struggling with the door, and ran forward to help her open it.

"Oh my god, thanks," the woman said as Maggie gallantly held the door open and then followed her in behind it.

The two women waited silently for the elevator, and when it came Maggie was dismayed to see a fob reader next to the buttons. She started patting her pockets and rifling through her bag, sighing exasperatedly as the other woman looked on.

"Shit, I must have left it at the hospital," Maggie muttered breathlessly. *Maggie, you're a natural,* said Frank over her shoulder.

"No worries, I gotchu," the woman replied, setting her bags down to produce a key fob that activated the buttons. "What floor?"

"Um, five, please." The woman pushed the button for the fifth floor, then (Maggie noted with relief) the third floor for herself.

"Thanks," said Maggie with an apologetic shrug. "Night shift, you know? I'd leave my head behind if it weren't attached." This additional play-acting wasn't needed as the elevator was already moving up, and Maggie may have been hamming it up for Frank's benefit at this point.

That's my girl, he said.

"Can't wait to hit the hay," Maggie added with a rub of her eyes.

We'll make a private eye of you yet.

The woman didn't respond, just nodded and smiled, and got off on the third floor.

At floor five, Maggie stepped off and looked down the hallway, trying to orient herself. She was last here six months ago, recently enough that her memory would be good except that she'd been reasonably drunk when she'd followed Al back here from a nearby bar. She closed her eyes to try to picture it, feeling Frank's impatient eyes upon her as she stood in quiet contemplation, trying to imagine where her feet had taken her on that disorienting night. *Five Oh Three,* was a voice that came to her, Al's voice this time, a memory. *Like the area code.*

We're in business, Frank, Maggie said silently as she opened her eyes and walked the short distance to door 503. She paused on arrival. *Now what,* she asked Frank. According to her watch it was 6:00 AM, certainly a controversial time to knock on a door unexpectedly. From the end of the hallway, Maggie's peripheral vision caught a camera's red action light blinking in observation. She tried to act casual, rifling through her bag again in theatrical search of a key that would never be found for the benefit of the camera, all the while listening for signs of life inside the apartment. Was that a shower running? She raised her hand up to the door to consider knocking, but couldn't pull the trigger, instead placing her palm on the door as a faith healer might do. What if Al's in there? What if she's not? But what if she is?

Through the peephole, Maggie could sense some movement on the other side of the door, shadows passing that briefly obscured the light. Shocked out of her stasis, she rapped her knuckles politely on the door, in that pattern for shave-and-a-haircut that for some reason signifies friendliness.

There was a click from the door as the lock was turned over, and Maggie took a step back as the door swung open. A young woman, early 20s maybe, with long blonde hair, stood there with her eyebrows raised, and Maggie immediately started apologizing, while Frank interjected loudly in her ear.

"Oh, gosh, I'm so sorry I must have the wrong apartment," Maggie started to say, while she heard from over her shoulder, *no apologies during an investigation, try again.* "Unless, um. You don't happen to know Al Power, do you?"

The woman rolled her eyes. "You mean my deadbeat landlord? Yeah, I'd sure like to know where she is." *She knows more than she thinks she knows.*

"Oh? Are you renting from her?"

"Yeah, I've been renting this condo from her for four months and the bathroom sink has been dripping the whole damn time. Jokes on her though, because I ain't paying the water bill, she is. Can't imagine why she won't just get a plumber out here, it's gotta be hundreds of dollars down the damn drain."

"Have you talked with her about it?"

The woman looked askance at Maggie. "And who the fuck are you, exactly?" Maggie had forgotten that the special dispensation for questioning, granted to her as a doctor, didn't extend to early morning door-knocks with strangers.

"Oh, gosh, I'm sorry. I should have introduced myself. I'm —"

Frank piped in just before Maggie could make a terrible mistake. *Not the truth, Owens, anything but the truth.*

"I'm Dr. Owens with the Oregon Medical Board. We have an open investigation with Dr. Power, and it's important that we reach her." Maggie could feel Frank beaming with pride, even if she couldn't see him.

The woman took on a knowing nod, and her body language softened. "I had heard a rumor about that, you know. She did seem to need to get out of here in a hurry."

Maggie sucked in her cheeks just slightly to steady her face. "It's a very serious matter, you see. Do you have any contact information for Dr. Power? A place where you're sending rent? Phone, forwarding address, anything like that?"

"Yeah, I *wish* I had a forwarding address. I keep getting her stupid junk mail. My rent comes out through automated bill pay, so I can't really help you there other than it keeps comin' out. I've got a phone number she never answers, an email that keeps gettin' bounced. Where ever she is, she's leavin' me alone for now, so whatever."

"Ah, I see, well that's certainly helpful." *The mail, Mags, get the mail.* "Have you been saving the mail? I am in contact with Dr. Powers' family, and they've been receiving her correspondence."

The woman smiled a big smile in relief and shut the door for a second. When she returned, she had a stack of envelopes, brochures, and magazines, all addressed to Dr. Alice Power. "Here you go, good riddance."

Maggie accepted the pile of mail, wondering at the same time if she had just committed a federal crime of some kind. *You're not an investigator if you haven't tampered with the mail at least once,* Frank assured her. *Feds don't care, they're doin' it too.* The paper felt good against her fingers, tangible.

"Thank you, miss — I'm sorry, I don't think I caught your name."

"I didn't tell you my name. Whatever this lady's got herself involved in got nothin' to do with me."

"Sure, of course, I understand," Maggie said. "Can I give you my number to pass on? Just in case Dr. Power gets in touch with you?"

The nameless woman shrugged. "Be my guest. I ain't got no paper, though."

Maggie tore a strip of paper from one of the envelopes she'd just been handed, dug a pen out from her bag and wrote her phone number in block lettering, along with *Dr. Florence Owens, Oregon Medical Board, Senior Investigator.*

At least a few of those words were true. Owens, Medical, Investigator. Was impersonating a Medical Board officer another crime? She'd have to worry about that another day.

After the woman closed the door, Maggie felt her watch buzz.

Shit. It was 6:30, and she was due at the hospital in fifteen minutes. She'd be joining resident rounds that morning. Even with the excitement of this new lead, the thought of being late caused her jaw to clench and her heart rate to rise perceptibly. *C'mon Frank, we got real work to do,* she said as she speed-walked toward the stairwell. On the way down, she summoned an Uber on her phone, happy for the excuse to skirt the tram ride.

As she skipped down the stairs, she stuffed the pile of mail into her bag, popping up the collar on her jacket. *Whaddya think about that, Frank? Our first evidence,* she said, patting the bag and its ill-gotten contents. As she burst out the front door of the Daniel, she added: *because I deserve it.*

With three minutes until the arrival of her Uber, Maggie had just enough time to smoke half a cigarette on the corner, which she did with purpose and direction. The morning sun was shining on her face. *I deserve it,* she thought again.

Maggie's destination for the morning was the Green Team workroom, the Green Team being her assigned allegiance in the *Risk*-inspired color wars that made up Portland University Hospital's Internal Medicine structure. Each team had an assigned group of attending physicians, along with residents, interns, and a parade of medical students who would float in and out. These allegiances were usually made for life, and when she was set to return, the Department Chair, a graying statue of a man with the memory of an elephant, had said to her, "Green Team, right?" as if it were plainly obvious just by looking at her. A Green Team attending might, because of ill call or vacation trade or poor planning, be assigned to cover the Red Team or Yellow Team or Blue Team for a day, but they will not feel the warm welcome of inside jokes and secret snack stashes that one feels with their home team. They will, on the other hand, be talked about unkindly after their departure, like *can you believe Dr. Owens follows the SPRINT trial* or conversely, *can you believe Dr. Owens doesn't follow the SPRINT trial,* depending on the team's position on a particular controversy. *Yeah, Red Team isn't as evidence-based as Green Team,* they might say, *I'm so glad I got assigned here.*

The Green Team workroom was strategically located in the geographic center of the old hospital building, flanked to the east and the west and the north and the south by nursing stations and patient rooms, as far from the exit doors as they could have made it, like a cocoon, or a trap. The room was devoid of windows, something it had in common with a Las Vegas casino and other places where time is a meaningless construct. A hotel bar. An ant colony. The Green Team Workroom's official room number was 667, which always made Maggie laugh, knowing that the rooms on either side of this one were 665 and 668, *and we know what room it is, really.* She had spent twelve to sixteen hours a day there for several months in medical school, and though the halls had been remodeled in the same manner as the rest of the hospital, the path to get there returned to her like that of a winter goose returning to its sunny southern home. A feeling of safety entered her body on the path, and her muscles relaxed.

When she reached the end of the patient ward and turned the corner into the cul-de-sac that held the Green Team Workroom on its end, the door stood in shadow under a fluorescent bulb that had been burned out since before Maggie had even been in medical school.

The door, still wooden and opaque and cluttered with papers, stood in stark disorganized contrast to the other sleek and remodeled glass and wood-veneered doors on the ward, as if it were a vintage home that a benevolent remodeling-tornado had skipped over in tearing its path of restoration through the corridor. This was the fate of every resident workroom, as far as Maggie could tell; medical residents, deprived of sleep and good sense as they were, always seemed to clutter the threshold or their spaces with a psychotic collage of sentimental debris that only made sense in context to its inhabitants.

In this case: A picture of a dog in a superman costume, thought bubble saying, "Green Team to the Rescue," subtle fart drawn out the dog's back end. Calligraphic sign reminding everyone to Dance Like No One Is Watching, but Dance had been scratched out and replaced with Replete Electrolytes. Handmade certificate reading "World's Highest Lactate," with a tourniquet tied into a makeshift blue ribbon and stapled in the corner. And so on. Like a clubhouse, to which the admission fee was a bargain at only 50% of your excess telomeres amortized over four years. So it is, and so it always shall be.

Maggie stood in front of the door for a moment, looking to see if any of her own tags from years-ago had still remained. She was half-squatted checking out a custom bumper sticker on the door that said, "Green Team Residents Do It With Contrast" when the door swung open, and she stood up suddenly in surprise. The weight of her messenger bag caught her to one side, and she found herself toppling out of her Danskos, catching herself on the wall just in time to avoid splaying out on the faux-wood-grain flooring. She heard a laugh and looked up to find a tall, curly-haired and oddly familiar man staring at her bemusedly with a hand on the now-open door.

"Ah! You must be Dr. Owens," said the man, who had *Dr. J. Miller, Internal Medicine* stitched on a wrinkled white coat. Maggie nodded but forgot to respond, as she was searching her brain for how she knew this man. Had they gone to school together?

"You're trying to figure out where you know me," he said with a sparkle in his eye, as Maggie remounted her shoes. Maggie nodded again, mouth hanging just a little open, one eyebrow raised. "I'm kind of famous on KnockKnock," he said faux-modestly. "Dancindoctorjack? That's me. I'm Jack." With his statement he broke into a kind of burlesque dance that involved faux-suggestive pulls on the stethoscope around his neck, followed by a turnaround where he faced away from her, looked back over his shoulder, and did a brief ass-shimmy. He turned back around and took stock of her face again, obviously hoping this had been a Big Reveal. Behind Jack, Maggie could see a couple of residents looking on at their interaction and actively rolling their eyes.

Maggie shook her head. "I'm not on KnockKnock, sorry. But I'm sure we've met. Did you ever work in Missouri, by any chance?"

"No, I — oh!" Jack smiled broadly, revealing veneered and whitened teeth that briefly dazzled Maggie. He said in a sing-song voice, "I know where we know each other."

"Oh, yeah?"

Jack lowered his voice into a whisper. "Does '*Colloid in the streets, crystalline in the sheets*' ring a bell to you?"

Maggie's face took on that of a deer who has just become aware of its fate, glassy and distant. Jack was, of course, quoting her *p*Value* profile back at her. The reason she'd seen Jack before was they'd matched just yesterday.

Maggie gave him a *don't you dare* look, glancing at the residents to see if they'd heard this. "Wait, did you say you're Dancin' Doctor Jack? From KnockKnock? On second thought, that *is* probably where I know you," she said, just a little louder than she needed to. "So nice to meet you."

"Welcome to the Green Team. Come on in," Jack said, moving aside now and opening the door all the way to allow entry. "Have a seat somewhere. I have a quick meeting I have to take but should be back in a bit to get you oriented. Rounds will start in thirty minutes." Maggie nodded and ducked through the door.

The door opened on a scene that was so familiar to Maggie; it was as if she'd walked through a portal into her own past life, except her coat was a little longer and the computers were (only a little) nicer. One (assumed post-call) resident was passed out napping on a plaid-upholstered couch, sunken into a resident-shaped indentation in the worn fabric, towel slung over his eyes. Another resident was slumped over in a corner cubicle, speaking low and fast into a dictation handset. A brown-haired resident with a tousled ponytail was shoving a bowl of oatmeal into her mouth while scanning through a dog-eared textbook and making notes on a sign-out sheet she had folded into a kind of medical origami that allowed for maximal note-space. A forgotten pager was beeping intermittently in a bag somewhere, and the coat hooks were hung not with clothing but with stray stethoscopes awaiting the return of their owners from the night shift. Piles of printed paper articles on management of hyponatremia and differentiation of types of renal failure were scattered carelessly on every surface. A whiteboard was scrawled with the hieroglyphic phrase QSOFA at the top, and unintelligible numeric chicken scratch underneath. Mismatched and half-broken office chairs, arranged around a central table that itself was adorned with mismatched snacks. Assorted Clif and Luna Bars in a wicker basket, next to several open packages of novelty Oreos, flanked by a donut box with only a single undesirable cake donut remaining behind for a time of desperation, adjacent to a pile of browning and neglected bananas.

Not looking up from her oatmeal, the tousled-ponytail greeted her with a warning.

"Don't open the fridge. Collin found maggots growing in the freezer compartment this morning. Someone left some ice cream in there, but it melted."

"Yeah," another resident said, "that fridge hasn't really kept anything cold in a while. I guess we should have stopped putting food in it, heh."

The other resident shrugged his shoulders up like what're you gonna do, smiling apologetically at Maggie, adding, "It's not much, but it's home. I'm Henry, by the way. I'm an intern. Collin's over on the couch, sleeping off his night shift." Henry held out a hand to shake hers, and Maggie tried to remember how to confidently shake it back, handshakes having been *verboten* for long enough that she'd gotten out of the habit.

"Maggie Owens, I'm a new attending. I'll be on next week. Just shadowing today."

The tousled ponytail looked up from her oatmeal and smiled at their guest. "And I'm Olive. Third year. Welcome to the Jungle." She held out her hand as well.

Maggie smiled. "The Jungle, huh? Do you have fun and games?"

The ponytail gave her a confused look. "Um. . .what?"

Maggie was taken aback. "You know, like the Guns N' Roses song? Wasn't that what you were referencing?"

Olive shook her head, explaining that The Jungle was an Upton Sinclair reference, of course. "You know, because of the maggots." Olive gestured to the refrigerator in question. "Do you want to meet them? We were thinking we could train them like a flea circus."

Maggie had long ago gotten out of the shared-hospital-refrigerator game, not being eager to join any kind of custodial agreement for cleaning/defrosting and upkeep, but actual maggots seemed a little beyond the pale. After all, this now maggot-hatchery was still co-located within the workroom, threatening at any moment to lose its seal and pop open, spilling its seething maggot-load onto the floor. On the other hand, maggots having made a comeback in the care of necrotic wounds, perhaps this could come in handy in a pinch?

Maggie, nose wrinkled reflexively, wasn't sure what to say, so what she did say was, "No, thank you, though. Kind of you to offer." She could feel her face contorting in disgust, so she tried to cover it up by grabbing a lemon-flavored Luna Bar. She suppressed her nausea and half-listened as Collin regaled Olive with tales of recent medical wizardry. *Have you worked with Doctor Salt yet? Boy, is he amazing — he diagnosed an aortic regurgitation by looking at this guy's uvula. His uvula? Yes. But can't you just get an echo? But that's not the point, Olive, his UVULA.* And so on.

In parallel, Maggie's worried mind quietly riffed on the activities of the nearby refrigerator-maggots, as they slowly consumed the entrails of melted ice cream (from which they had not spontaneously generated, Maggie knew, which meant that fly eggs had been somehow present in the ice cream during manufacture, ew). Maybe some of the maggots would become flies, and these flies — sealed in the sarcophagus of the refrigerator — would await one of a number of fates, which Maggie began to imagine vividly.

First, Maggie imagined the fruit flies starving to death, becoming thinner and thinner as their little fly eyes bugged out in the process, as the stronger surviving flies ate the dead carcasses of their peers, as they merged into one massive, cannibalistic super fly who eventually had no further fuel to keep on going. How long would that take, she wondered, years? Perhaps the refrigerator would be destined to fail first, as she imagined the melting mass of ice cream eventually breaching the gates of its container, causing a catastrophic short-circuit to the refrigeration motor, after which all flies would burn up in a firestorm, along with the Green Team Workroom itself. Perhaps larger forces would win out, though, as one day the sea level would surely rise above the level of the resident workroom, and the refrigerator and its maggot-residents would be swept away in a Great Flood, thus freeing them to breed once again in the now-water-logged grave of humanity. Maggie saw herself swept away in this same flood, gasping for air above water-level, getting a mouthful of fruit flies instead.

None of the imagined fates involved the residents or hospital properly disposing of the refrigerator and replacing it with a new unit, as this seemed terribly unlikely.

Maggie knew a few things about the life cycle of a fruit fly. In her younger and more idealistic days, at her midwestern state school, Maggie had co-authored a Student Treatise on Insect Euthanasia, which sought to reduce the suffering of *Drosophila* flies in the University laboratories where they were used to study genetic inheritance. The laboratories' habit of freezing the flies and then drowning them in ethanol came into great concern in this document, as did the premise itself of breeding *Drosophila* families in increasingly mutant perturbations. Sure, the magnitude of each fly was small, and perhaps the suffering of one was measured in picograms and milliseconds, but as a shear percentage of the flies' tiny lives, multiplied by the volume of tiny fly bodies that suffered this fate, et cetera et cetera. This treatise debated the various avenues for suffering of the tiny *Drosophila* body, the likelihood of various levels of sentience to clock that suffering, and the putative mechanisms for alleviating it. It weighed the practicality of utilizing tiny injections of potassium chloride (hyper-caffeinated college students being unlikely to possess such fine motor skill to reliably hit the thoracic ganglia of a fruit fly, it was determined), isoflurane gas anesthesia followed by mechanical crushing (the preferred method of the authors, though prohibitively expensive given the safety regulations needed for hyper-caffeinated and presumably stoned college students to have access to gas anesthesia), carbon dioxide asphyxiation (effective, but time-consuming, and unclear if the excited behavior exhibited just prior to death was a sign of fly euphoria or fly suffering). There was the option of humane release, though *Drosophila* being largely indoor creatures and the Midwest being relatively cold in the winter, at that point you may as well freeze them yourself, the laboratory director had pointed out. Unless you were suggesting we release them into your own apartment to cohabitate peacefully forever, said the laboratory director, which absolutely no one was.

In the end, in spite of the picketing and less-than-civil debate that tended to mark college ethical controversies, to this day, as far as Maggie knew, the flies were still frozen and drowned in ethanol. So it was, and so it shall always be. It had seemed astonishingly important at the time. Maggie was considering the practicality of obtaining some isoflurane gas to release within the doomed refrigerator when Frank flicked her on the back of the neck, causing her to startle.

Owens, get your head out of your ass and do something useful. Frank had no use for theoretical treatises on fruit fly suffering. Frank was a man of action. *Al didn't not die so you could sit here worrying about some goddamn flies.*

Frank was right, of course.

Maggie took out her phone and checked her call history again. The history confirmed her memory of what had happened. She had called a dead woman, and the dead woman had called her back. She opened up her text message thread to Al's number.

What message to send a ghost or zombie or bot or no one at all? She typed and erased a few possibilities. The stakes somehow couldn't be lower, if Al was indeed dead, but also felt impossibly high. *U up?*

No, no. *Long time no see.* No. *Thumbs up if you're alive, thumbs down if you're dead.* She settled on sending a photo of the Pink Floyd triangle with the rainbow prism passing through it, with a comment below that said: *In case you find yourself on the dark side of the moon.* She pressed send, saw the text arrive as blue to confirm that an iPhone, somewhere, had received this message, and then stared for a second more. She couldn't believe this was the first time she'd thought of this *dark side of the moon* pun. Would it be clever enough to pull Al out of hiding? If Al were dead, would the Al-replacing phone-robot that had called her this morning clock the double entendre about the moon? Her contemplation was broken as the word *Sent* below the image turned to the word *Read,* and she gasped out loud. Olive looked over at her briefly before returning to her oatmeal. Maggie gave an apologetic look and cast her eyes back down, just in time to see this:

. . .

Three dots appeared in the line below her message. The dots hung there for a moment, then disappeared. Maggie held her breath.

. . .

They appeared again. *Must be a long response,* Maggie thought, her skin electric with anticipation.

Al ain't dead, said Frank, *do you believe me now?*

Was it just that simple? Or was it something else? Were the dots the reflex of a spam bot, working up the nerve to send her a *bit.ly* link asking her to upgrade her car warranty or buy a timeshare property or invest in cryptocurrency? Or was it Al herself, searching for just the right *gif* to send back, scrolling past *Parking in the Rear* and *Brown-Eyed Girl* animations to ultimately choose the one of Homer Simpson sinking slyly back into the bushes?

No such *gif* appeared, just the dots, promising something but delivering nothing. Maggie thought about sending another message, but what could she say without feeling like a lunatic? *U dead, bro?*

Incoming, Frank said, and Maggie looked up just in time to see

Jack plopping his body into the chair next to her, clapping her on the back as he sat down, as if he were her high school football coach. She set her phone face down, but a thread still stretched from her mind's eye to the three dots, hanging there in suspense like beads of sweat that could drop at any moment as she willed them to hold on.

"Welcome to the Green Team, Dr. Owens," Jack said, holding out his hand to shake hers while giving a brief wink.

"Oh, welcome *back*, you mean. I was actually born in the Green Team, back when I myself was a baby doctor." Medical students are referred to in these diminutive terms. *Baby doctor. Scut monkey. Hey you.* "Couldn't stay away."

"Well, welcome *back*, then." Jack had a sly smile on his face that Maggie was trying not to see. "Did you happen to leave some ice cream in the freezer?"

"Maggot-flavored by any chance? I've been missing it."

"Well, it's been waiting for you. I think it's finally ready." Jack's eyebrows waggled up and down, and Maggie quickly changed the subject.

"So, what's changed in the last ten years? Catch me up."

"Right, right, of course. Gotta job to do. Let's pull up a computer. You used MaX before?"

Maggie looked over at Jack to see if he was serious, and he immediately cracked up. Obviously, Maggie had used MaX before; that was the joke. MaX had a near-monopoly on electronic medical records, thanks to the company's early habit of buying all the other start-ups, until its software language took up a full quadrant of every healthcare worker's brain.

"Okay, joking aside, have you used *this* version? The influx of billionaire money has got us the Cadillac, with AI decision support, predictive text, the *works*. Ambient scribe is coming soon, too. You should open up the Playground and mess around, you'll see."

Maggie did as she was asked, clicking on a merry-go-round-shaped icon on her desktop labeled MaX Playground. The Playground is where new doctors go to become indoctrinated into the language of The System, and also where errant doctors go to do penance for their mistakes, to be forgiven for their variances as they forgive those who cause variances against them. Where fake patients with names like Donald Duck and ZZZtest FakePatient could suffer the slings and arrows of technophobic errors without consequences in the corporeal realm. Where bioinformatics deities, from the clay of their own minds, could create endless human analogs with, one has to imagine, the wonderment and hilarity of God Himself. The universities might have been churning out programmers who hoped to design video games or program SpaceX Adventures, but all the money was in health care, and this was the result; the Playground had become an overwrought medically themed LARP analog.

In this case, The Playground opened up to a too-literal visual representation of an actual playground that was meant to evoke a certain sense of whimsy. *Ooh lookie, a slide for Admissions and a merry-go-round for Discharge Planning, perhaps this work task will be fun after all. I was going to go home to my family, but perhaps I'll check out these Order Entry monkey bars, that looks fun.* On one hand, annoyingly juvenile. On the other hand, what was the alternative? A blue screen with blocky white text? Whatever UX designer was responsible for this monstrosity, they had a family, they had hopes and dreams, they had career aspirations that certainly went beyond torturing stuffy doctors with childish conceits. And yet, here was Maggie, an adult with a doctoral degree, facing a decision between a swing set and a splash pad.

Maggie chose Splash Pad. The screen zoomed in on the splash pad briefly for effect before opening into a module meant to train her on fluid management in the hospital. She was greeted with a patient list themed for fish and waterfowl: Goose, Grey. Dick, Moby. Bob, Sponge. And so on. In the Playground, these aqueous dwellers perched precariously forever in a limbo that required either the addition or subtraction of some fluids from their digital bodies. These unfortunates existed only for the sake of mistakes; mistakes to be created over and over and over and over again before being reset to zero.

Maggie had a tendency to over-empathize with these imaginary patients, fretting endlessly over their fake problems as if they might feel real pain. Today, though, Maggie's mind drifted out of even this fantasy world and into another. She was imagining Al's phone, sitting atop a nightstand somewhere, buzzing with a dozen missed call notifications and a weird Pink Floyd text message. She briefly glanced back at her watch, which provided her no evidence that the call had been returned. She pictured Al's dead and rotting body clutching the phone, bones rattling with the buzzing of each incoming call, intermittently pushing the declination button just by vibratory happenstance. She pictured Al's limp and lifeless body being propped up in an operating room by a series of nurses who were maintaining for some reason the ruse that she was alive, laughing at the Pink Floyd *gif* as they puppeteered Al's mummified limbs through a hernia repair. She pictured Al alive, retired on some beach in Acapulco, having successfully fooled everyone into thinking she was dead. She did not, could not, picture some mundane reality in which she was just gone from this earth. That seemed too, too unlikely to be real.

Realizing she hadn't blinked in a full minute, Maggie closed her eyes tightly, rubbed them for a moment, and cleared her head.

"You know, if you subscribe to my KnockKnock channel, you can check out my Dot Phrase Discotheque Dance. It's got the most views," Jack said to her in the background.

"Oh, I see," said Maggie, snapping to and choosing *Goose, Grey* from the top of the fake patient list. The patient's profile popped up. It was, of course, a picture of a goose, dressed in a suit and tie.

Who is this chucklefuck? asked Frank, referring to either Jack or to Mr. Goose. Mr. Goose was a 62-year-old male, admitted for the chief complaint of dehydration. Mr. Goose had the following listed problems:

Dehydration, occupational, mild, unrelated to Alaskan Salmon Fishing.

Abnormality of cervical spine, not related to trauma, sequelae.

Bird bite, uncertain whether intentional, first occurrence.

Vocal cord dysfunction, congenital.

Poor Mr. Goose, burdened with these joke problems for the bemusement of some bored humans. Here he was, trapped in a reality where his thirst would be forever unquenchable, his dehydrated state existing not just here for Maggie in this moment but for dozens of other doctors trapped in this same training purgatory, all over the MaX empire. Even though she would and could fill him with fluids, restoring his renal function and his urinary output, the satisfaction would not last as it did for humans. For Mr. Goose, the moment Maggie logged out and walked away, MaX would return his theoretic goose body to its baseline state: sunken goose eyes, thready goose pulse, pale goose flesh, like a toddler without object permanence. Maggie could relate. Poor, poor Mr. Goose. She worked through his scenario quickly as MaX automated a number of helpful suggestions (fluid bolus, electrolyte corrections, monitoring for input and output), chiming each time she made the correct choice with a brief, twirling sound that sent a pleasurable shiver down her spine.

"You know, I'm nominated for a Webby Award this year," said Jack, apropos of nothing.

"Oh, I see, that's excellent," said Maggie, clicking on the second patient, whose name was *Bob, Sponge* and came with the profile photo to match. In this world, however, Mr. Bob was not an actual sponge under the sea, but rather a 54-year-old farmer admitted with a chief complaint of nausea and vomiting.

Can't fool me, farmer, Maggie thought.

Maggie had known some farmers in her life. When they showed up in board questions and in an emergency room or on a hospital ward, you could bet on it being Very Bad. Aortic dissection, myocardial infarction, ruptured aneurysm, end stage metastatic cancer of unknown primary. These were the types of things that could separate a farmer from the faithful completion of his agricultural duties. A farmer does not have panic attacks. A farmer does not have heartburn. A farmer does not have low back pain. A farmer does not have time for that shit. A farmer wakes up at 4 AM to run combines through dirt and stick his hand up a cow's ass. Until he drops dead in your waiting room.

MaX's suggestions popped up about as fast as Maggie could accept them; troponin-EKG-lactate (presuming a heart attack), chest xray (for an aortic dissection), metabolic panel, urinalysis, approve, approve, approve. The pleasing sound continued to fire every time she clicked an order, the happy chime of machine and human in agreement. Yes to the chest Xray, chime! Yes to the lactate, chime! Yes to the blood count and the aspirin and the hep lock. Chime! Chime! Chime! It was a recognizable sound, Maggie realized, the same one also used in a Las Vegas slot machine, or in that old Mario game when the little guy was collecting coins. She delighted in it, even knowing it was conditioning her. Then, in this sea of yes and more yes, Maggie stopped cold in her tracks at the next suggestion: an order for normal saline, bolus rate 999mL/hr, continuous, no end point. Sitting like a bomb, daring Maggie to defuse it. She stared directly into the camera atop the computer. That fluid rate was rarely advisable, but especially not for a farmer having a heart attack. Perhaps this was the point, Maggie thought. Just like real humans, given enough power and rope, an advanced AI was prone to fashion a noose with which they could encourage you to hang yourself.

Can't fool me, robot, Maggie thought as she rejected the saline order. Were it real fluid given to a real man, it would certainly have filled his most likely mid-heart-attack lungs with fluid, guaranteeing a gruesome flash pulmonary edema death from which he would not be resuscitated. Maggie imagined Mr. Bob, weathered and tanned hands having spent a lifetime working the land, with wrinkles now swelling and flattening with fluid engorgement, flesh increasingly edematous, breathing more and more labored and wet. *No machines,* Mr. Bob would insist. *I don't want any machines. Just let me go.* His skin would be weeping, soaking his bed sheets with saline sweat as his long-suffering farm wife looked on, her rugged ag-man succumbing to a flood that his failing heart-pump could no longer contain, the death of a thousand milliliters. *Make sure to feed the cows when you get home,* he would say, right before the lights went out.

Not today, robot. Maggie rejected the saline order, getting the chime that told her this was the right call. Keep this faux-farmer dry, that's his natural state anyhow. A fake cath lab was alerted, with hypothetical ins and outs to be closely tracked and replaced PRN to achieve net zero. Done.

Maggie had to admit, the feeling of fixing these machine patients was nearly as good as (maybe even better than, if she was forced to admit the truth), fixing the real ones. The real ones don't give you a nice chime at the end. The real ones only bitch at you about how many times a day you've ordered lab draws and ask why you're forcing them to eat a renal diet.

You sure do know how to make these machines happy, said Frank. *Is that what they're teachin' in doctor school these days?* Maggie couldn't see him, of course, but she felt Frank was probably taking a big drag off a Lucky Strike as he said this, and she felt a pang of jealousy.

"Pretty neat, huh?" Jack was looking over her shoulder and leaning into her in a way that allowed her to smell the Altoid on his breath. She wondered if he could clock her tobacco-smoke perfume in return, hoped he could.

"Yeah, I guess so." Truth was, no one particularly liked this system, but the forces that were motivated to change it were tired and busy from caring for patients, and the forces that profited from it were well-rested and drinking espresso from well-appointed offices, and so the system remained. The system was producing health care, wasn't it?

"Not that you'll need to do much with it. Most of the attending physicians just let the residents do all the ordering and whatnot. They're way faster at it anyhow. There's no reason for us to get too much into the weeds."

Olive, who had been listening in from the workstation next to them, piped in. "You know that's called weaponized incompetence, Dr. Miller."

"Not in a hospital, it's not. It's called *learning.*"

Maggie piped in, stirring the pot slightly. "Did you know, Dr. Miller, that some hospitals don't even *have* residents, and the attending has to do everything?"

Jack shuddered. "Maggie, Maggie, Maggie. I think those are just called nursing homes." Jack was leaning back in his chair, and had his feet kicked up on the desk in the universal sign of a man in charge. "Don't tell me you came from such a place."

Maggie nodded. "Sure did. County hospital in Missouri. Jackson County Memorial, maybe you've heard of it?"

If a record had been available in the room, it would have scratched itself to fill the sudden silence that fell. This mic drop would continue to work for another three to six months, when the number of hospital incidents would have piled up to a point where no one would even notice them by their individual names.

After a minute, Olive broke the silence. "*Shit*, Dr. Owens, glad you're here," she said, while Henry and Jack both made faces she supposed were trying to look sympathetic. Maggie broke the silence.

"Anyhow, rest assured some attendings do know how to put in orders and write H&Ps."

Olive pumped a fist in the air, chanting: "One of us! One of us!"

Jacks scoffed. "Oh, if the resident union gets their way, we'll be back there, eventually. You know we have to do in-house night shifts now? Attending physicians, sleeping in the hospital overnight, pshaw, as if working night shift alone isn't when you get *made* as a doctor." Jack was using the word *made* in much the same way as Maggie had seen done in mafia movies, an apt reference. "I mean, how are you supposed to learn to swim if you don't get thrown into the deep end?"

Olive gave Jack a dagger-look. "I don't know, maybe by taking swimming lessons and slowly building confidence as the water gets deeper?"

"Ugh, *as if.* You want medical training to last thirty years? Because that's how you get medical training that lasts thirty years. By going slow and sleeping eight hours a night like a *baby*."

So it is and so it always has been, the older doctors bemoaning how the younger ones *have it so easy* while the younger doctors are drowning and drowning and drowning, everyone looking for a younger or weaker entity that they can stand upon to stay afloat. Maggie sighed, thinking of Christopher, back in Missouri, working unending night shifts without complaining, picking up extras to cover when Maggie had started to have panic attacks before work, coming in early to relieve one of their practice partners who was pregnant. Somehow, all of that over-the-top kindness had just made things worse for Maggie, for it had only heightened her own sense of failure.

Maggie's wrist buzzed with an incoming message, and she sat up straight with a start, feeling the thrill of possibility for just a moment, but her face fell when she saw who the message was from. DoCTR Debbie had sent her the following:

Hey! Just want to check in about a little problem! Looks like someone named Frank T. Blood signed for your spot in computer lab yesterday, so we can't give you credit for the onboarding. Oopsie! Please come by this afternoon to sign the attestation so we can keep you active!

HaHAHAHA! Frank was now beside himself with glee. *Looks like ol' Frank Blood is still gettin' some credit in this world! Hoo boy, looks like you got yourself a real pickle! HaHAha!*

Maggie frowned, deleted the message, and was rescued by Jack as he stood up and raised his baritone voice above the din.

"Alright team, time for rounds!" He clapped loudly a few times to rally the group, a move that awakened the sleeping couch-resident who briefly groaned before turning back over. Jack lowered his voice to give Maggie an aside. "You gotta keep a tight leash on this group; it's like herding cats around here." He raised his voice again for the group:

"Who's got the highest floor today?" Olive piped up.

"I've got someone on Fourteen."

"We have a winner. We start on Fourteen today." Jack walked to the door to open it before gesturing for Henry to lead the way through. Maggie grabbed her messenger bag and slung it over her shoulder, reluctant to separate herself from her smokes or Al's mail in these uncertain times.

As they all filed out of the room, Maggie noticed a full-color photo of a middle-aged white man hanging above the door, a philandering billionaire whose ex-wife had just endowed the hospital with a billion dollars as a thanks for treating her cancer. The residents were reaching up and tapping the photo as they passed through. Above the photo was a hand-printed post-it that said, "FROM HIS BILLIONS, OUR STRENGTH."

Jack continued holding the door as the residents' brisk walking pace took them just out of earshot, and as Maggie went to pass last through the door, Jack placed his hand on her arm, subtly stopping her in her tracks as he leaned in and spoke in a low, conspiratorial tone, "You know what floor that *really* is, don't you? The fourteenth floor?" Maggie knew there was officially no thirteenth floor in a hospital. Not officially. And so the Fourteenth was, you know. Maggie shrugged and nodded.

"Yeah, of course I know."

Jack's hand remained on her back for longer than necessary, until Maggie jutted an elbow out and moved her body away from his, turning back and saying as she walked away, "You should know, I don't shit where I eat."

This wasn't true, of course, but it felt good to say it. Before Jack could respond, Maggie turned forward and double-timed her steps to catch up with the rest of the team, who were nearing an elevator bank at the end of the hall.

"Stairs, people! We start the day with STAIRS!" Jack clapped again at the group from behind, and they groaned collectively and moved laterally to the stairwell door. "Elevators are for weenies and losers!" Frank, who Maggie could tell was leaning against the wall with his fedora pulled low over his eyes in a classic private eye stance, let out a low whistle.

I don't suppose you're gonna let this Mickey Mouse motherfucker call you a weenie, are you?

Maggie caught up to the group as Jack lagged behind, distracted by something on his phone, and she shuffled with them through the door into the stairwell. She let the heavy door shut behind her, then brought her voice into a whisper and held her finger to her lips. "Follow me, I've got a trick for this," she said in an insistent whisper, as she headed *down* the stairs instead of up, the confused group following her out of pure instinct. "We'll go down a floor to lose him and then take the elevator up and beat him there."

"Now we're talking!" said Olive. "Now we're talking."

"*Viva la revolution!*" said Henry dramatically as he charged down the stairs behind their new fearless leader.

"I've never felt more alive!" said the medical student, who remained nameless.

Maggie held open the 5th floor door as the group shuffled through and Maggie shut the door gingerly behind her just as she heard Jack's lumbering long strides come through the door above. She spied through the narrow window as Jack headed up the stairway two-at-a-time, none the wiser.

The system is a maze, and if you play your cards right, you can sometimes, sometimes, get the cheese at the end instead of the shock.

Revolution, my ass, said Frank, correctly.

It's not a revolution, said Maggie silently back to him, *but it's something. It's something.* The elevator pinged its arrival, and she strode into it with a smug smile, crossing her arms as the doors closed and she was pulled comfortably up to the top, heart rate stable at 65. She pulled the phone out again, checking for messages, checking the status of the three dots. There were no messages, there were no dots. There were no more calls. But somewhere out there — somewhere out there, there was something happening. She wasn't sure what, but it was something.

Chapter 8

MS3

It was the third year of medical school, and Maggie was scrolling. Her cursor reached the end of the page, and there was a brief pause, and then new material appeared, and she scrolled again. This repeated and repeated and repeated. She was unsure how long she'd been at it, ten minutes or twenty or an hour, and she kept thinking she should stop, but she couldn't.

"This patient hasn't had normal potassium in *two years,*" she said to the room. "How is that possible?" The room did not respond. "They keep getting admitted for low potassium, but no one seems to care *why.*"

If the first year of medical school is a baptism into medicine, when the students are submerged in the blessed waters of the River Hippocrates for rebirth; the third year is when they emerge on the banks covered in the slime and the muck and the feces of Actual Medicine. The third year is when they become privy to the fact that the baptism site is downstream from a sewage treatment plant, and that this is also their drinking water. The third year is when they are finally tasked with the care of actual human bodies who are not yet dead but could be, if you aren't careful.

So here was Maggie, in her third year of medical school, trying to solve the mystery of one man's missing potassium, and she was scrolling and scrolling to look for evidence. It was six AM, and Maggie was sitting in the Green Team workroom, wrestling with years of lab results for her patient, an eighty-year-old nursing home resident who had been sent in by his facility after having passed out on his way to the restroom for the third time that week. The first two times they hadn't called, but the third time they thought to bring him in. Maggie tried to make sense of the patterns of low potassiums and high sodiums and low blood pressures and elevated heart rates that should make sense, but just didn't. When she had tried to graph them, the medical record had produced something that looked like a starburst of colors and vectors heading off in all directions. So now she was scrolling, thinking if she could just reach the bottom, she might reach some Sentinel Event that would explain it all.

Christopher sat at the next workstation, often on rotation with Maggie as the alphabetic distribution of the students had continued on into third year. He was doing something similar but for a younger patient, and with social work notes instead of lab results.

"Can you believe last time they just discharged this patient with open wounds on his legs to the street? *To the street.*" He shook his head. "We gotta do better."

"Hey guys, get a load of Saint Christopher over here," came a heckling voice from a workstation on the other side of the room. "Patron saint of frequent flyers."

"Give it a rest, Al," Christopher responded. "You can feel free to not give a shit, but somebody needs to." He returned his scrolling, replacing any further commentary with loud sighs. Maggie glanced over with worry, tapping him gently on the arm to break him from this misery.

She leaned over to him, speaking softly, hoping Al wouldn't hear over the Taylor Swift *Red* album that was playing on her computer speakers.

"*Ohmygosh,*" she said, as if it were a thought that just happened to strike her in that moment. "I just remembered! I read something about a new risk score for predicting necrotizing fasciitis. Maybe you could calculate it to present on rounds!" Enthusiastic, but not too directive. "I know it's silly," she said, knowing that it was not at all silly, it was the opposite of silly, it was dead fucking serious, "but I'll bet Dr. Marshall would love it."

Christopher looked over at Maggie, who was widening her eyes to look as much like an innocent baby otter as possible, and smiled. "Thanks, yeah, that's a good idea."

"I, um. I printed out the article for you," Maggie added, eyelashes batting wildly, shoulders curved forward to make her body small, unobtrusive, unobjectionable. "In case you want it."

"Cool, cool. Thanks. Cool. Yeah, great." Christopher accepted the paper from her hand with the enthusiasm of one who has just been gifted by a process server. He laid it aside and continued his tour of past social work notes. "What does it matter if we can't find him housing and he bounces right back? That's what I want to know."

Al chimed in from across the room. "You know what will solve his housing problems? If he dies of *nec fasc.*"

The last bit was pronounced as *neck fash*, a bit of shorthand slang that identified Al as being in the secret club of medically trained talkers who no longer had to say full words. People who drew little fishbone-shaped shibboleths filled with numbers on scraps of paper, the way the early Christians drew the Jesus fish symbol in the dirt, to signal silently to others that *I'm one of you.*

"That man needs a scalpel before he needs anything else," Al added. "Cutting is curing, you know?"

Christopher let out an extended breath and rubbed his face in his hands. "I'm going to go grab some water while we're waiting on the residents to get back." He gave Maggie's shoulder a quick squeeze as he stood up, as a gesture of conciliation. "Give me your bottle, I'll fill you up, too." Maggie handed him a bone dry Nalgene bottle that had been gathering dust beside her workstation for more than a day, giving him a quiet *thanks, babe* that she hoped wouldn't register to Al.

Al turned around as Christopher walked out of the door and out of earshot. "You know he's a lost cause, right?" she asked. Maggie swung around in her chair, seeing Al leaned back casually, looking over with a bemused smile on her face. "Dude should've gone to social work school, not med school."

"Maybe I'm the one who's a lost cause, you never know. Maybe we all are. Maybe he's the only one who understands the assignment." Al was making intense eye contact with Maggie as she said this, and Maggie was making it back. Al finally got to the point.

"So you guys are like, still together?" Al had a single eyebrow raised, a countenance that Maggie could not have matched even if she tried. Maggie nodded affirmation.

"Huh," said Al. "You gonna couples match?"

Maggie tilted her head and smiled, raising both eyebrows. "What's it to you?"

"I mean, if you're going to sleep your way into something, at least sleep your way into the top instead of the middle." Maggie shrugged and returned to scrolling.

"I tried, Al. The top wasn't interested." Al laughed, mission accomplished, and Maggie turned serious. "Besides, not every relationship is transactional, you know? Not everybody needs to sleep their way *into* something."

"Ok, sure, but are you really going to couples-match with someone who barely passed Step 1?"

Maggie's smile finally fell. Al was relaying a true reality of medicine — that intra-student love affairs were not just condoned during medical education, they were actually baked into the career pathway that took them from their general medical education into the required specialty training of residency.

Before graduation, every medical student enters something called *The Match*, a hyper-competitive multi-interview leap of faith in which students and residency programs spend a few months speed dating and then ranking each other in order of preference, before a cold and impersonal (and omniscient and infallible and wise) computer algorithm spits out (hopefully) the destination at which all these new doctors will spend the next 3-7 years of their life working 40 to 80 (or who are we kidding probably 100) hours a week for little to no pay. In *couples matching*, students opt to tie their fate to that of their sexual partner; one of the few job offers that is extended to you, at least in part, based on the value of whoever it is you are fucking.

Couples matching is saying to your parter, *I like you enough to live in Duluth, Minnesota for 3 to 7 years if it comes to that.* Couples matching is having to say *I'm sorry* every day for the rest of your life, if you are a *hard worker who showed improvement* and your partner is a *once in a lifetime medical intellect.* Couples matching is either not for the faint of heart, or only for the faint of heart, depending on your perspective.

Maggie knew that, she *knew* that what medical student didn't know that? She also knew that every oocyte in her body had been there since the day she was born, and that the attrition of those eggs was proceeding at a rate that did not care if she might match at a Top Ten medicine program if she played her cards right, did not care that she still had five-to-seven years before she could realistically plan to take twelve weeks off for maternity leave anyhow. She was riding a centripetal carnival ride that combined the slingshot of career possibility with the downward slide of female fertility, and sometimes wasn't it okay to choose something comfortable and ordinary like someone who fetches you water and makes sure you eat lunch? And wouldn't these comforts keep her sane through the desert landscape of residency?

"Christopher's going to be a great doctor," said Maggie, "and I don't give a shit about board scores," she added, as a person who cared a great many shits about board scores, because they provided the objective measure of her self-worth she had always craved. "Anyhow, you may not shit where you eat, but I find it to be very convenient."

Maggie turned back around to her screen and the potassium. Al smiled and raised her hands in surrender, just in time for Christopher to return to the room with full water bottles.

"Maybe I can convince this resident to order an ACTH level," Maggie said aloud, scrolling and scrolling and scrolling, as if this were what was on her mind in his absence.

Christopher sat down next to Maggie, pushed a water bottle her way, picked up the article from next to his computer, and started reading, glancing over at her to give a quick smile and a thumbs-up as he did so. Maggie picked up the water, taking a long drink from the bottle as she looked back at Christopher, trying to feel the cool satisfaction of the water as it went down as fully as she could. The water was good for her, of course it was. So, so, so *good*.

The potassium guy would die later that day, and Maggie would cry, thinking *if she just had one more day*.

"Then *what*," her supervising resident would say to her tears. "Everybody you ever take care of is going to die, Maggie. You know that, right? You just move on to the next."

This is the education of a doctor, more than the names of the parts, how to keep going.

CHAPTER 9

Maggie had to admit, as she shuffled through the hospital with the Green Team, that she had missed the rhythm of an academic hospital, with its collision of entourages and big personalities all jockeying for attention. In medical school she'd assigned soundtracks to the constant channel-changing of rotations, when her life was a radio stuck in seeking mode. Surgery service had been a late 90s ska revival, choppy and frenetic. Intensive Care was brooding and focused techno, with the hiss of ventilators keeping time in the background like Nine Inch Nails' *Closer*. Pediatrics, smiling in the face of the hardest and least-compensated job in medicine, cheerfully sang along to the soundtrack of the newest Disney movie. In training she thought her life would always be like that, but once Maggie was an attending she'd suddenly been a lone trumpet melody, wailing out into the night. They don't tell you how lonely you can be, in this place where you are surrounded by people, if you aren't traveling with a crew. People look right past you until they need something from you. Even people who are married to you.

Maggie had expected Internal Medicine rounds to be what she'd remembered from her training — plodding, ethereal, like those circumferential Enya tracks about saving the whales. Internists are famous for stalling progress with probing lines of inquiry fired at learners who stand shifting their weight on aching and unslept feet. They might say, apropos of very little, *tell me what are the 8 most common causes of metabolic acidosis* followed by *and the difference between proximal and distal renal tubular acidosis* and then *but what is type IV renal tubular acidosis* and *yes but which exchange transporter is affected* on and on and on until the student or resident has come to the realization that they are nothing, they will never be anything, and they have no hope except possibly to read more. Maggie would never admit it, but she was looking forward to being the one in power in this equation, for once in her life.

Jack, though, was one of those other types of Internal Medicine doctors, a rare but vocal subset who felt it was important to teach the students and residents *how it's really done,* a type of doctor more about the ends than the means.

Rounds started with him hitting a timer on his watch with a flourish. "Olive, you have three minutes, no more," he said, before settling in to swipe at his phone.

"Three minutes? Even for FUO?" Olive queried with a hint of desperation.

"*Especially* for FUO. *Especially,*" Jack replied, not raising his eyes from his phone.

Fever of Unknown Origin (abbreviated FUO, a purposeful reference to its flighted counterpart) came with a sense of *Unsolved Mysteries* secret fun that every doctor knows about even if they rarely say it out loud. That part of the doctor-brain that releases dopamine in the course of puzzle-solving loves FUO, which by necessity involves a thorough and invasive patient history (*Any foreign travel? Sexual partners? Substance use? Pet parrots?*) and a guns-blazing approach to the ordering of tests.

Olive reported the following: *Patient denies any travel outside the United States or to Florida or Texas. He has had no exposure to armadillos or turtles he is aware of. He denies exposure to well water or consumption of freshwater from streams or rivers. He does not drink unpasteurized milk. He denies intravenous drug use or any exposure to stimulants or other unusual substances. He has one sexual partner who is a cis-woman. As far as he knows, this relationship is monogamous.*

Patient denies. As far as he knows. A doctor remains skeptical. A doctor does not actually visit the patient's home like Dr. House on television does, but oh boy does a doctor want to. A doctor reports the patient's statements of denial, while ordering the HIV test and the urine drug screen and the tuberculosis test. The tests are an outright admission to the patient that you have considered they could be lying. *Just to make sure we aren't missing anything, you understand.* And because the patient is wearing a cheap floral gown that is open in the back and laying in a hospital bed, and you are standing over the edge of the bed wearing a long coat and you are flanked by a (Fecolith? Borborygmus?) of students and residents, the patient says *yes of course I understand you have to do your job, which is to assume I am lying to you at all times until objective evidence proves otherwise.*

You never believe the official story, said Frank, *not for a minute,* as he watched the scene play out. Frank was picking the dirt out from under his nails with a pocket-knife. *Not for a single, god-damn minute.* Was Frank talking about the patient or about Alice, or did it matter? He was right either way.

Maggie's watch buzzed, and her heart skipped.

Until she looked, the message could still be from Al, inviting Maggie to meet her in Bora Bora, and not a reminder to breathe or a congratulatory message for standing or one of the other mundane bombardments her watch would send her hourly. Maggie imagined Al on the beach with a prosthetic nose and a long blonde wig blowing in the breeze, sipping on a comically oversized coconut-shell cocktail. If she never looked, Al could stay that way forever. So, she didn't look. Olive continued on: *His sedimentation rate is over 100 which rules out malingering.*

Malingering. Secondary gain. Conversion disorder. An unspoken urine drug screen. A well-placed set of quotation marks in the history and physical. Mostly patients tell the truth, but the language remains. *The patient denies.*

Was MaX also being trained with this skepticism, in preparation for the day it took over her job entirely? Or would it take everything the patient told it at face value, gullible at its core? Is this ability to consider half-truths thus an essential part of our humanity?

Maggie's wrist buzzed again, and she looked this time. *SocialEyes notification.*

Maggie's eyes lit up and she gasped, loud enough that Olive paused in her differential between *Adult Onset Still's Disease* and *Endocarditis*, and Maggie had to smile apologetically and wave her on.

Maggie took her phone out with a sense of purpose, a furrowed brow and a nod that would suggest she was pulling up a clinical review article on Brucellosis rather than a social media site. The act wasn't necessary, of course, as Maggie's estimation of how much attention anyone might pay to her always was outsized to the reality. Still, it felt good to keep up an appearance, if even for herself. She opened the app with eyes squinted, trying to blur out the actual front-page content while still spying the inbox flag in the top corner where — indeed — a new message awaited her. It was from Elizabeth. With everything that had happened that morning, Maggie forgot she'd sent her a message yesterday.

Elizabeth had sent her regards, saying *we missed you at the reunion*, and then offered contact info for Alice's brother. *I'm sure he'd love to hear from someone who had good memories of her.* The name of Al's brother was Brian Power, which was exactly the kind of thing someone might make up in a pinch. Maggie looked up just in time for Jack to cut off Olive's presentation and usher people into the room.

"Three minutes is up! Tighten it up, Olive, you're using too many words today. We're just gonna pan-scan him, right? Hopefully that was the plan that you were *eventually* going to get to. What's this dude's name again? Williams?"

Olive nodded, and Maggie slipped her phone back in her pocket. Jack looked at his watch and shook his head before rubbing his face in exasperation.

The group formed a line to hit the hand sanitizer before filing into Mr. Williams' room. Jack breezed past it and took his position at the foot of Mr. Williams' bed, clasping his hands in front of his waist as the rest of his group arranged themselves behind him in the flying-V formation that always seems to manifest on academic rounds.

"Good morning, sir, how was your night?" Jack did not introduce himself, but his name was embroidered on a long white coat, and his title was visible in his silver-streaked hair and strong jaw, and this was enough of an introduction.

"Nice to finally meet my doctor," Mr. Williams said with a congenial smile, looking at his watch, implying perhaps that Jack had just returned from an early round of golf or a leisurely breakfast. "Did the nurse tell you all my secrets?" Mr. Williams gestured at Olive when he said the word *nurse*. "I'll admit I've never had a date ask me about armadillos before" — he paused either for laughs or to take a breath — "but I'll answer any questions" — stopping for another breath — "if it helps you to figure out what's making me sick."

Jack held a hand out and rested it on the footboard, patting it as if this act might provide some comfort to the man.

"Don't you worry, sir. I suspect we'll have this figured out by the end of the day. We're going to send you down for a CT scan from soup to nuts" — he held one hand to his chin and one to his groin when he said this — "and I suspect we'll find something. In the meantime, we've started some antibiotics just to be sure."

"Sounds like a plan," Mr. Williams said, adding after a short breath, "boss."

Maggie noticed something in the cadence of his speech and leaned close to Olive's ear. "*Chest Xray,*" she whispered.

"*Looked clear,*" Olive whispered back, shrugging, but understanding what Maggie was getting at. Maggie nodded.

Frank, who had been leaning against the back wall of the room, turning a toothpick in his teeth, took the opportunity to pipe up. *That's a man got something eatin' him up inside. I should know, right? I ain't talking' about a tapeworm, either. I'm talkin' about a FIRE inside 'im. I ain't no doctor, but I know a dead man when I see one.*

Jack wrapped up quickly with a flourish of his stethoscope on the man's chest, declaring things to be *clear as a bell* before heading back through the pack of students and residents and toward the door. Maggie reached a hand out to stop him briefly as he walked by.

"Hey, Olive and I are going to hang back a minute. We'll catch up with you. I have a few physical exam teachings I'd like to do." Jack shrugged, waved a hand toward the bed to say *be my guest*, and walked out. After Jack was gone, Maggie sidled up to the side of the bed and sat on the rolling stool that had been stowed there for this purpose. Olive crouched on the other side of the bed, without the benefit of the stool, but with the benefit of young knees that hadn't yet begun the predictable deterioration that had caused Maggie to groan slightly as she sat.

"Mr. Williams, I'm Dr. Owens, I'm one of the attending physicians here." Mr. Williams not-subtly glanced at her badge to confirm this credential.

"Nice to meet you, ma'am." He reached a hand out and shook Maggie's hand firmly.

"Mind if I check some things out? Sometimes it's helpful before we do the pan scan, to know where to look on the pictures."

"No problem, ma'am."

"May I?" she asked, gesturing to look at his hand, which was now resting upon the top of his coarse hospital blanket.

"No problem," he said, offering his hand to Maggie without hesitation. "If you must hold my hand, I won't stop you."

The whole bed was undulating with the inflation and deflation cycles of a hospital air mattress, cycles that were meant to constantly redistribute the pressure points that accumulate when one doesn't leave the bed for days on end. The hissing, clunking mechanism that did that inflating and deflating was loud, rhythmic, like a heartbeat, and Maggie found it loud enough that she had to lean in close to Mr. Williams to hear him over the din, with his voice weakened by illness.

Maggie inspected the nails, noticing a roundness to them that made her furrow a brow. The fingertips can be a surprising window into the state of a person's health, with nails that crack or whiten under certain vitamin deficiencies, tiny vessels that pulse under the nail bed when a heart valve is leaky. In this case, Maggie saw the signs of sudden bone growth under the surface of the finger tips, a sign called *clubbing* that often harkened to a certain kind of problem in the lungs.

"Mr. Williams, I know you've already been asked this, and I ask only out of medical need, you must understand, but have you at any time used an IV drug, even just one time?" Mr. Williams broke into a broad smile, threw his head back and laughed a big laugh, one that made him grab his stomach with the hand not being held by Maggie.

"Sorry to laugh, ma'am, but no, I'm not a drug user. I do volunteer at a shelter downtown, though, so I guess I coulda been exposed."

"Shelter?" Maggie placed his hand back on the bed, looking at Olive, whose expression made it clear she hadn't gleaned this piece of data in her history.

"Yeah, a place for youth, lot of teenagers whose parents kicked them out, you know how it is. I play basketball with them every Wednesday. Mostly they kick my ass."

"Well," said Maggie, "that's very kind of you."

"Nah," he said. "I get more out of it than the kids, to be honest. It's the least I can do in a world like this, right? Started during the pandemic just to have a reason to leave the house."

You're right, he's a dead man for sure, Maggie said to Frank, who chuckled a pompous *told you so* under his breath.

"What was that?" Mr. Williams said to Maggie. "I didn't catch that."

Had she said that out loud? Maggie looked over at Olive, who had a shocked look on her face.

"I said, you're a good man, Mr. Williams. You're a good man." She patted him on the hand again, and Mr. Williams beamed back at her.

"You think I'll be outta here by Wednesday?"

Nice people die, Maggie thought, *and mean people live forever.* This is an immutable law of medicine, one that a doctor learns over and over and over again in their career.

"Well, we can certainly hope so," Maggie said, technically not lying. "Is it okay if I listen to your heart?" Maggie held her stethoscope up as if to make clear that it was a literal heart to which she would listen, rather than some existential-emotional state of being.

"You think you'll hear something that the doctor didn't?" The phrasing of this statement made it clear Mr. Williams had already forgotten the words *doctor* and *physician* with which Maggie had introduced herself.

"I might, you never know!"

He's a dead man, anyway, why make him feel bad? Just move on. Maggie laid her stethoscope to his chest, slipping the bell just under the top of his gown, gently resting the other hand against his shoulder to provide the counter pressure that allowed a subtle expansion of the bell that would improve the capture of certain sounds. She pulled it back off after a second and glanced at Olive.

"Olive, all I could hear when I listened was the air compressor from the mattress, was that what you heard too?" This was a question and also a judgment. Olive looked down at the floor and nodded. "OK if I turn this off for a minute?" Maggie asked, at the same time as she reached to pull a plug out from the wall. "It'll help us to hear."

As the bed-motor spun down into an inert silence, the strange quiet seemed to amplify every sound in the room, and Maggie found she was holding her own breath as she listened. Olive followed suit. The two kneeled on either side of the bed, hands against the chest of this semi-clad man they had only just met, Maggie with brow furrowed and Olive with eyebrows raised; their respective concentration-faces revealing something about their orientation to the world in general.

"Time was, I would have paid good money to have two women kneeling next to my bed like this." Mr. Williams chuckled, looking around for another man in the room who might laugh with him, finding only Maggie shushing him and pointing to the stethoscope that had amplified this crude statement into her ears. Mr. Williams couldn't see or hear him, but Frank cracked up from the corner, saying *tell me about it, buddy. You just wait until she decides she's gotta get her hands on your deep dorsal vein, you won't be laughin' then, hoo boy.*

Maggie smiled, but she didn't laugh. *You're a dead man, anyway, Mr. Williams,* she thought, *so you might as well get your laughs in now.*

The impulse for the infirm to become amateur stand-up comics is understandable. They may not realize it so explicitly, but when your body is put in this vulnerable state — prostrate before an unending line of standing white-coated people carrying needles and asking too-personal questions and touching your bare chest with only a moments notice and getting intimate knowledge of your inner workings of a kind that you cannot access yourself, and using code words to describe your shortcomings right in front of you — in this type of vulnerability, it can only seem fair to make a joke about blow jobs as a doctor kneels next to your bed or say *won't you at least take me to dinner first* as a nurse inserts a urinary catheter or *don't tell my wife we've got to stop meeting like this* as if the phlebotomist coming in for a blood draw was here for an illicit and unusual affair and not a tiny assault on your bodily integrity. There is a reason people make these jokes comparing the intimate insults of medicine to other, more pleasurable acts of intimacy. It transports people, for just a moment, from the panic and the drudgery and the pain of their current situation, into something lighter, less consequential, an imagined world in which perhaps the CT scans and the bone marrow biopsies and the chemotherapy might all be an elaborate hyper-realistic setup for a porno shoot. We all do this type of imagining in times of stress, don't we? Maggie had stopped being bothered by it years ago. Maggie caught Olive's eyes in the aftermath of this statement, rolling her eyes and shrugging as if to tell her, *what're you gonna do amirite?*

This is the education a young doctor gets, as much as the medicine, how to build up their armor when faced with the slings and arrows of human nature. This is the system that builds a doctor, and these were doctors, weren't they? Weren't they?

Maggie let out the breath she had been holding, removed her stethoscope, and looked over at Mr. Williams, staying low to the ground to avoid towering too much. From this angle, she could see the quickened pulse bounding in his neck, and could sense more easily the extra labor in his breath.

"Can I push on your stomach, sir?"

"Please do," said Mr. Williams.

Maggie put her hands on the spot that she'd seen Mr. Williams holding earlier, on the lower left side, looking subtly at his mouth while she did it.

"Does that hurt?"

"No, no, nothing like that," he said, but his lips tightened a bit, and his breath became more shallow. Maggie pushed her hands a little deeper and noticed his nostrils flare a bit, but he still denied pain. Her hands moved in a circular motion she'd learned for deeper palpation, and stopped when her fingers caught the borders of something firm and foreign that had been hiding in the soup of intestines. Mr. Williams' eyes widened and he let out a small cough.

Maggie gave Mr. Williams a knowing look, and he looked away quickly.

"No pain, I promise," he said. "I just gotta pee, is all."

Maggie put a hand on his arm, patting it as if he were a close friend, and Olive mirrored her on the other side. "Of course, Mr. Williams," Maggie said. *You're a dead man, anyhow, so I'll forgive you.*

Maggie's cruel reverie was broken by a manic beep that jarred her ears from above, as the IV pump screeched a warning that its feeder bag was empty. The sound was in a high register with just a hint of electronic vocal fry, designed to be insistent and un-ignorable, as if the end of a dose of antibiotics were an emergency on par with a hungry baby trapped in a house fire. This alarm was designed by people who severely underestimated the level of noxious pain that could be ignored by a tired nurse juggling twelve high-acuity patients at the end of a double shift. It was close enough to Maggie's ear, though, that her hand reached back and mashed at the largest and most red button she could find, in the same annoyed reflex arc that had once hit the snooze button for an 8am college calculus class.

"Oh thank god," Mr. Williams said as the sound stopped. "Last night they let it go for thirty minutes." Maggie showed him the button in question and gave him the authority to press it when he needed to.

"Goddamn, that's the most useful thing anyone has done for me all day," Mr. Williams said, as Maggie stood to regard the label on the deflated bag.

"Fluids?" She looked over at Olive, who was looking at her notes.

"Yeah, his lactate was a little high."

Lactate, Maggie knew, goes up when there is tissue that is not getting enough blood flow to keep the cells alive. Sometimes this means dehydration, and you give fluids. Sometimes this means infection, and you give antibiotics. Sometimes you're not sure, and so you give both. And sometimes it is neither, and the lactate is simply a harbinger of doom.

I told you, said Frank, *I told you, that there is something DEAD inside this man. Take it from one who KNOWS.*

"Oh," Maggie said, trying not to give away any emotion, "very good. Try to get some rest, Mr. Williams," Maggie said. *Not that you'll need it where you're going,* she added silently for Frank's benefit.

Maggie and Olive left the room (*whaddya say we have a second date tomorrow,* said Mr. Williams jokingly on their way out, and the two women politely laughed), and reconvened at a workstation down the hall.

"I'm pretty sure that man has colon cancer," Maggie said to Olive when they were out of earshot. "I'm guessing metastatic."

"What?" Olive had included *occult neoplasm* on her differential, but fairly low down, below even *Bubonic Plague* and *Extrapulmonary Tuberculosis.*

"Don't you think it's gotta be infectious? What with the shelter volunteer work and all?" Olive saw the shelter as an infectious disease risk, an exposure that could mark an entry point for something exotic and interesting. Maggie, though, knew better.

"Nice people die," Maggie said to Olive, with the same tone with which she might impart knowledge of how to dose penicillin or how to read an EKG. "It's the law of nature."

"Oh," said Olive, "I hadn't thought of that."

Later in this day, Olive would receive results of the pan scan of this man's body, results that will show a *probable large mass in the descending colon,* along with tiny shotgun pellets of metastasis into his liver and his lungs, little time bombs that were large enough to subtly affect his breath, but too small to show up obviously on the initial chest Xray. When Maggie hears the news, she'll feel a perverse pride in having been right, followed by an immediate guilt at having taken pleasure in being right about something so terrible. What use is guilt, though? The laws of the universe are what they are. She did not build the system, the system has built her.

Olive's pager went off with a message from Jack: *We're on the 12ᵗʰ floor when you're done playing in the sandbox.*

"You go ahead," Maggie said. "I'll catch up to you in a bit. I've got a couple emails I need to send."

Olive scuttled off, and Maggie sat behind a workstation and watched her disappear. When Olive was out of sight, Maggie added aloud, "You too, Frank. I'll catch up to you later. I need to be alone for a minute."

Frank's boots clicked down the hallway and out of earshot.

Maggie waited a minute, then walked down to the stairwell and pushed through its door. On the other side, she sat on the top step, pulled out her phone, and found the SocialEyes message with Alice's brother's contact information on it. The cold of the concrete penetrated the thick fabric of her white coat as she sat and sent a shiver up her spine as she stared at the name: Brian Power. Brian Power. She felt it was a name she would have remembered. She tried to imagine Al referencing a brother, as they sat typing notes on Christmas Eve during their third year. Had she?

Plans for Christmas? Al had asked as Maggie calculated the potassium deficit of a fluid-bloated diabetic. *No, you?* Maggie had said back, but then her memory of that evening went into a dark hole of millimoles and milliequivalents and total body water and ideal body weight and sodium corrections. She could remember the potassium in question was 2.1, but no further details of their family holiday talk.

She did have some other memories of that December. She could remember Al had bought her a Mt. Vesuvius Christmas ornament (where she had found such a thing, Maggie still wondered), slipping it into her white coat pocket furtively in the workroom while Christopher hadn't been looking, along with a Post-It that said *Careful, this shit's about to blow.* Maggie had, in turn, bought Al a bumper sticker from a local novelty store with a picture of the Earth and *Don't Shit Where You Eat* written across it, which she had tucked into Al's *Sabatine's Pocket Medicine* guide right before rounds. Al had found it just before presenting on a septic cellulitis patient, and had laughed that laugh that made Maggie feel accomplished, and Maggie had been beaming and giddy for the rest of the day. Christopher had asked Maggie about it later and she had lied, knowing that it wasn't cheating but it wasn't innocent either.

Maggie stared back at the name *Brian Power*. Having a brother with that name seemed like the type of thing Al would have mentioned in all of her name talk, and Maggie was now certain she'd never heard it. Al's father was named Oliver Power, Maggie remembered this, it was memorable. But no brother's name. No mother's name either, for that matter. How close had they been that Maggie had no idea about her family? It had been Al's choice not to talk about them, surely, but also Maggie hadn't really asked. Maggie realized she'd assumed Al was estranged from them, but had no real data to back that up.

Well, here goes nothing, she thought, as she composed a message to this Brian Power. She started and erased and started again, trying to find the right tone. A tone that would be correct if it were directed to the brother of a dead woman, but that might also be correct if this Brian Power were the secret *nom de plume* of an actually alive Al playing a prank. *Hey there.* Delete. *Hello!* Delete. *Dear Brian.* No. *Hi Brian -* that'll work. *I am so sorry to bother you.* Try again, don't assume bother. *I know this message might be unexpected.* Not quite right. *I hope I'm not bothering you —* there it was — *but I was a friend and a classmate of your sister, Alice. I was sorry to hear —* no, *I have regrettably just learned of her death —*no, not that word, too direct — *I was saddened to learn of her passing. I have been thinking of her and wonder if you might be willing to talk to me. I will understand if the answer is no. Sincerely —* delete — *Warmly, Maggie.* Or maybe, *Maggie Owens.* Or what about, *Yours, Dr. Maggie Owens.* Maggie put her phone number at the bottom, assuming this Brian Power to be a person of her own generation who still called people on telephone numbers.

Maggie checked her text message thread one last time, noting again the word *Read* was really there under her message, but the three dots were now gone. She put her phone back in her pocket, stood, and descended the stairs to the 12th floor.

Maggie rejoined the Green Team on the 12th floor, as rounds circled down by gravity through the clockwise stairwell-drain of the hospital building, stopping on each floor to either add or subtract fluid and electrolytes from the bodies of the people contained within, the achievement of a net state of Fluid Zero being the ultimate goal of any Medicine team. Jack kept the team moving efficiently and pointedly, giving the occasional *sotto voce* aside to Maggie as the team walked ahead but not exactly out of earshot. *You've got to watch Henry, he has a tendency toward premature closure if you know what I mean hahaha. Olive's a strong resident, but a little overconfident, if you ask me. I wish Collin would learn to keep his subjective and objective separate, you know?* Maggie noticed how the resident in question would slow their pace just a bit as Jack spoke, closing the gap between them to one that was definitely within an audible range, and how Jack would seem to just keep talking, if anything, a little louder. Perhaps this was the form that feedback took on the team, indirect and with plausible deniability. This is the system that makes a doctor.

Maggie's watch buzzed again as Henry presented on a 25-year-old online influencer with cyclic vomiting syndrome who had been admitted for symptom management.

Message from: Brian Power

Hot diggity dog, we caught a fish, Frank said, having apparently returned from whatever cat nap he had gone off to. Maggie took a deep breath and looked over at Jack, who was looking down at his phone, swiping and doing a muted little dance to himself as Henry spoke. She looked at Henry, who was looking at Jack swiping, and carrying on with his presentation. *This is her seventeenth admission this year for electrolyte abnormalities related to vomiting,* he was saying, *and she has requested that we consider port placement to allow for home management of fluids.*

Jack put his phone down and frowned, motioning to the team to stay put while he ducked into the room. Maggie could hear his one-sided conversation from the hallway, as Jack spoke in an uninterruptible string of declarations.

Hey sweetheart good morning I'm Dr. Miller attending physician and the plan for today is to get you tanked up okay, and psych is going to see you okay to see if they can help you out but the fluids can go in a regular IV and I don't think you'll be here long okay great see you later let your nurse know if you need more nausea meds okay take care pleasure to meet you.

Jack emerged with a satisfied smile, looking at his own watch as if to confirm the speed record that he had just set for himself before looking at the team with the well-recognizable face of a confident man, a face that said *that's how it's done people.* This is the education of a doctor, as much as the memorizing of body parts and disease pathways and genetic variants. *How it's done.* Later, his chart notes would reflect a physical exam that did not require him to have come any closer than ten feet. *Generally alert and normocephalic skin well perfused and non-cyanotic no rash on exposed skin no visible edema*, it would say, all technically correct.

"Welp, managed to be done by ten-thirty, not bad, team! I wanna see notes done by noon conference, page me if you need anything." Jack brushed off the shoulders of his white coat as the group dispersed by category, the interns with quick steps in one direction, senior residents with slower steps in another, and the medical student left standing in the hallway alone to consider the life choices that had led them up to this moment.

Jack gestured to Maggie.

"Wanna grab some coffee and talk attending stuff? If there's time, I might record a new dance if you wanna see how the magic happens." He was already walking toward the stairwell as he said this, assuming her affirmation and forcing her to step in double time to catch up. Maggie pulled up alongside him, checked her watch theatrically, then looked over apologetically.

"Geez, I was hoping to spend a little more time with MaX, then I've gotta get up to DoCTR to sign some HR forms."

Jack scoffed. "Why don't you just work in the lounge? Computers are better there anyhow. I'm headed in that direction. Walk with me?" It wasn't really a question, but Maggie answered it by following him through the heavy door to the stairwell.

"Hey," Jack added, "team's wagering on fever guy's diagnosis, wanna pick a horse?" Jack pulled out a little notebook. "We got three votes for acute HIV, one for Cryptococcus, and two for Lupus."

"That's morbid," said Maggie.

"And?"

"Put me down for colon cancer with mets."

"Whoa, a bold move from the rookie! I like it." Jack put his note-book away and started taking the stairs two at a time.

"I'm hardly a rookie," said Maggie. "I have at least three gray hairs."

"Point taken, m'lady," said Jack, having clearly not taken the point. "So," he continued, "what's your deal?"

Maggie had been executing a controlled fall down the stairs to keep her Danksos on her feet while she tried to keep up with Jack's long legs.

Slow down, people, said Frank in her ear, having rejoined after rounds. *I ain't got skin on my feet to keep up this kinda pace.* Frank's Achilles tendons, having been severed, were flopping uselessly from side to side like pigtails as he tumbled down the stairs behind them. Maggie began to let her own shoes fall slowly and heavily on the concrete to try and audibly signal Jack to slow down.

"My deal?" *Kerthunk, kerthunk. Sigh.* "I'm not sure what you mean."

"I mean, what's your *deal*, you know? Word on the street is you got the highest board scores the department chair has ever seen. So what were you doing in *Missouri,* at a *county hospital?* And what are you doing *here?* Just here for the money?"

"Honestly," said Maggie, being legitimately honest, "it just seemed like the easiest place to go, back to where I was born. Like a salmon, or something."

"You came back to procreate and then die?" said Jack, turning around to grin at Maggie from several steps below her. "You should consider putting that on your *p*Value* profile."

"Not a bad idea," said Maggie.

They reached the third floor landing, and Jack opened the door and walked through, throwing the door open wide in his wake as an alternative to actually holding it for her. Down the hall, he repeated this as they walked through the door to the doctor's lounge, forcing Maggie to first duck out of the way of the swinging door, then run forward to catch it as it swung toward closed. By the time she collected herself and made it through the door, Jack had already grabbed his black coffee and was making his way back out.

"I'll catch you at noon conference, don't forget to sign your forms," he said as he passed by. "DoCTR doesn't fuck around in my experience." He didn't glance back, but rather held a hand above his head and gestured with a backward wave. Maggie saw his feet practicing a little two-step shuffle as he walked away.

The sign-in sheet. She had said this as an excuse, but maybe she should just run up and do it, shouldn't she? It would only take a minute. She was reluctant to leave the lounge, though; it seemed so peaceful here. In the late morning, the lounge had taken on the feel of a rock concert thirty minutes after the last encore, where there were ghosts of the party, but the party itself had moved on. The morning donuts were gone, save for that half a cake donut that always seemed to be Left Behind after the more righteous donuts had been raptured into hungry bellies. There was one lone unconsumed too-bruised banana and a sugar-free Yoplait shoved in the back corner of a cold holding table, and the Coca Cola sponsor-fridge was emptied of all products save the caffeine-free Diet. Across the room, a cardiologist was swiping right-right-right on a tablet of EKG images, while his other hand swiped left-left-left on an iPhone distractedly. Daytime tennis matches were playing to no one on the corner TV. A psychiatrist nodded off in the corner, loudly failing an impromptu sleep study, *honk-shoo, honk-shoo.* Maggie was tempted to join him.

Maggie perused the snack options, not even hungry, just out of habit. Eat when you can. Pee when you can, and so forth, survival instincts that fade over time but never extinguish. She snagged the sorry banana, always one to root for the underdog, noticing as she did a domed camera blinking at her from the ceiling above the snack tray with its infrared eye. This was the way of things, now. She wondered who was on the other side of that camera, and to what purpose. Keeping the fun-size yogurts safe from undeserving student fingers?

Observing the heaving shoulders of crying residents at 2 AM? Alerting the executive suite to the early signs of diminishing morale? *The doctors have stopped eating the bananas,* one exec might say, *do you think we should assign a wellness module?*

At least they're transparent about it, thought Maggie. The cameras could have easily been hidden, secretive. The size of a camera being what it was, the ceiling tiles being removable as they were, the walls being wired as walls were these days, the Money being as big as it was. The Suit puts a camera where the Suit wishes to put a camera. If they want eyes on you, the eyes are there. Maybe DoCTR Debbie was watching, Maggie thought, waiting for her to make her next move. Maggie hoped so.

Maggie stood next to the trash can to eat her banana, looking periodically up at the camera with a tiny smile. She made a deal with herself that she'd use her phone to hop on SocialEyes for just a minute, just long enough to read the reply from Alice's brother. Only as long as it took to eat the banana. Then she'd move on. She opened SocialEyes and took the first bite.

Message from: Brian Power.

I'm sorry to say I don't know much about my sister and probably can't give you anything useful. It's nice to know she had at least one friend. I'm sorry for your loss. Brian Power.

Maggie took another bite, chewing slowly as she considered this. *I don't know much about my sister.*

Neither did I, apparently. If this had been meant to squash Maggie's curiosity, it had backfired, as she was more curious than ever. *Sorry for your loss.* What an odd response from a sibling. As if Maggie were the one deserving of comfort and consideration. Maggie found herself circumspect, now taking smaller and smaller bites as the banana went on. She started to construct a reply. *I don't want to bother you but.* No, erase. *I'd still love to talk with you, I would find it very comforting.* She stared at those words. Would Brian Power feel compelled to comfort her? Was she a monster for wanting him to? If she could just manage to take these banana bites in half lives, could she eat this banana forever? She erased and reconsidered. *If you'd consider a brief conversation, please let me know. It would mean so much to me.* Her mouth finally reached that bit of banana-gristle at the end, and she had to admit that it was over. She pressed send and added the banana peel to the precarious top of the already-overstuffed trash can, and headed past the snoring psychiatrist to a back corner workstation.

Her intention was to sign right into MaX and do some more training modules, that was what she'd told herself was her intention, at least. She sat down at an empty cubicle and swiped a badge at the RFID on the side, and the screen lit up with recognition. *Hello, Maggie Owens.* Maggie wondered if DoCTR Debbie had just received a notification about her sign-in, if she was sitting somewhere with the forged sign-in-sheet in hand, clutching it in such a way as to wrinkle it in her grip, saying *I'm gonna get that Owens if it's the last thing I do.*

Frank sat beside her, saying *you know you don't solve a case by following the rules, Maggie. You solve a case by breaking 'em.*

"Be quiet, Frank," Maggie said softly, as she logged into MaX.

Shame, said Frank, *I thought you were more than this. Fortune favors the bold, or haven't you heard.*

Boldness means different things to different people. To Frank T. Blood, it might mean hitching onto the back of the Burlington Northern Santa Fe freight line as it barrels through the outskirts of St. Paul, Minnesota, hoping to lay eyes on a jewel thief who has hidden himself in a grain car. To Maggie, it might mean saying *fuck the sign-in sheet,* it might mean navigating right to SocialEyes, even knowing that somewhere, an IT guy or an HR minder might be watching you do it. The eye of a camera was mounted atop the monitor, after all, and it led to somewhere.

"Alright, Frank," Maggie said. "Alright."

Maggie winked at the camera and then navigated the browser to SocialEyes. A lesser institution would have just blocked such sites, could have forced Maggie's hand into completing her work out of pure boredom. But what's the fun in that? Blocking the websites would be a rookie mistake. *Not* blocking the sites, so that you can spy on the activity of your hospital's highly paid but overly lonely professionals — that is the Next Level Shit for a Suit. Somewhere in the terms of service, they have agreed to be monitored and then assumed that you won't follow through on it, but a Coat underestimates the vigor with which a Suit might gather ammo for a future fight. Ammo like *oh look the new girl who thinks she's so clever with her fake signature is on SocialEyes in the Doctor's Lounge, let's listen in.* From there, a Suit could watch this doctor on her med school's private class page, scrolling and scrolling until she reaches the time last year when someone named Alice Power had repeatedly and desperately asked her former classmates to send her money on CashApp to help with legal fees *because I know you motherfuckers have it.* Having done so, a Suit could then tap into the webcam, watching the darting of Maggie's eyeballs and the furrowing of her brow as Alice drunkenly rants about the State Medical Board and their obsession with the contents of her urine, suggesting that they plan to use it for the manufacture of a new kind of lesbian Premarin. *It would be funny if only.* More and more pleading for cash, *please guys, my career is on the line, my lawyer just needs another 10K for an expert witness.* Then one last message that simply said, *Sayonara, suckers.* Then, a few weeks later, the message from Elizabeth with comments underneath ranging from *how sad* to *I guess I won't be getting my money back*, under which a series of sub-comments debate the appropriateness of making such a comment about a dead person. If someone were indeed activating the webcam at her workstation, they would see the gathering of a tear on Maggie's left eye as she recalled how callous sometimes people in medicine could be about their own and each other's shortcomings.

You don't believe this shit, do you? Frank stood over her shoulder, indignantly blowing tobacco smoke into the confined space of the cubicle. *Because I sure fucking don't.*

"What's not to believe?" Maggie muttered quietly. "Seems pretty clear to me."

Circumstantial, Frank insisted. *Look at the evidence, why dontcha.* He eyed her messenger bag. *Look.*

"What evidence, Frank? What evi—"

The mail. Maggie had forgotten about it until now. She pulled the stack of paper out of her bag and laid it on the desk, her fingers brushing against her cigarette box in the act. *I'll tend to you later,* she said to the box, as her head started to ache just a little in wanting. *I promise.*

The mail was largely actual junk: a mailer advertising the opening of a new dental office, discount coupons for a local Mexican restaurant, a PUH alumni magazine that Maggie herself had received a few weeks ago and thrown directly in the recycling. She took time now with this ill-begotten copy, lingering on a glossy photo spread of Jack, in which he laid in a break-dancing repose across the centerfold under the headline, *Dancing Doctor Brings Joy in the Aftermath of Pandemic.* He wasn't bad to look at, Maggie had to admit, and had a certain over-polished kind of charm. In the back of the magazine, an *In Memorium* section gave a gushing retrospective about a recently departed cardiologist who had invented some kind of heart valve back in the day, along with a few more concise one or two-liners for relative nobody-doctors who had all died at reasonable old ages "after long battles" with a variety of cancers. Underneath this was a single, unadorned mention of Al.

Alice Power, MD, class of 2015, passed away at the age of 38.

No further information was offered, but the reader could draw their own conclusions, of course. A doctor who dies of cancer is a hero who gets flowery elisions about having been *a brave warrior to the end* or *called home to God.* A doctor who dies of their own fault does not get these things. They get the fewest words possible and are never spoken of again, under fear of it catching on as some kind of in-house contagion. *Don't want people trying to get out of their contracts the easy way,* somewhere a hospital administrator might have said. *They just don't make doctors like they used to. Perhaps we should throw a pizza party for morale,* someone might say while sitting at a long, mirror-finish table on a high floor of a downtown building. *Nah, maybe just a Thank You Healthcare Heroes banner for the entrance? Something cheery, with ClipArt of balloons on one end. Should we bring donuts back to the Doctor's Lounge? Maybe assign a Suicide Prevention Module in the Wellness Curriculum? Yes, yes of course.*

Maggie tossed the magazine aside and examined the last piece of mail, one she'd torn a strip from to leave her number with the nameless woman. A few dark rings of coffee stained both sides of the envelope, which had been used as a coaster. It was typewritten, addressed to Alice S. Power. Where the strip had been torn, a remnant of a return address remained:

Gold Beach, OR 97444

Looks official, she thought, noticing now she'd torn all the way through the letter as well in her haste to have something to write on. Thanks to the fold of the letter, the strip she'd torn managed to remove some of the top, bottom, and middle parts of the text. *Some detective I am,* she thought, smoothing the paper onto the table. The coffee had soaked through the paper enough to degrade the fibers and rendered some of the text lost to time. It was dated for three months ago, and read:

Confirmation of Employment

We are pleased to confirm your acceptance of the employment offer dated June 1-[unreadable]

Your Start Date is confirmed as July 2-[unreadable]

Please report to the address listed abo-[unreadable]

For questions about what to bring your first day , please call 541-6-[unreadable]

The remainder of the letter was missing, and the letterhead with the address hadn't survived the hasty tearing either, so her only lead was the portion of address that had remained on the envelope. *Gold Beach, OR? What kind of job would Al be taking all the way out there?* She set the letter aside and opened up a Google browser and typed in *Gold Beach, Oregon Jobs.*

Gold Beach was a sleepy town on the southern coast of Oregon, full of a mix of year-round retirees, seasonal tourists, and the remnants of a previously robust logging operation that still limped along abreast tightening environmental regulations. Based on the online listings, the most robust employer in the town was Curry General Hospital, a critical access hospital that offered a full complement of services to the aging and isolated coastal population. *Acute Care Nurse. Janitorial Services. Health Unit Coordinator. Family Medicine Physician. General Surgeon.*

Just as she was coming to an excited conclusion in her mind, as if by divine providence, she heard Jess' voice come over her shoulder.

"Hey, Mags, do you want to. . ." she started, but then got close enough to register Maggie's Google search results. "What, are you already looking for a new job? You just got here!"

Maggie quickly folded the paper and tucked it into white coat pocket before turning around.

"Jess. Jess. Jess. JESS." She couldn't quite formulate the words that she wanted to say, knowing that the content of them may come across as rightfully lunatic. "Jess," she took a deep breath and tried to calm her delivery, "Hear me out. . ." She paused, considering how best to word this. "Al's *alive*." Maggie paused, trying to fix her face to be calm and rational and believable. Jess pulled a chair over from a neighboring workstation and sat herself next to Maggie, giving a concerned face, or at least trying to.

"C'mon, Mags. I know it's hard to accept —"

"No, no, it's not like that. I have *evidence.*" Maggie gestured to her screen. "*You've gotta see this.*" Maggie pulled out her phone, taking Jess through the series of events of the last few days, sheepishly and apologetically explaining how she had called and texted Alice's old number, *no I'm not sure why I did it but look*, showing her the early morning call back, *how else do you explain this?* "I'm telling you, I just have this feeling that she's alive — I don't know, is it crazy to think maybe she faked it?" Jess tried to furrow her brow, succeeding only in moving her hairline a few millimeters lower.

"I don't know, Maggie. I feel like there must be some other explanation."

Maggie kept pushing, because if she could get Jess on board with her theory, it might take it out of the realm of *magical thinking* or *delusion* and into the realm of *Possibilities That Should Be Explored.*

"It's too many coincidences, Jess. There's gotta be a reason."

Maggie didn't mention the letter, which would have required her to fess up to breaking and entering and mail fraud, but she offered the possibility that Al just *wants* us to think she's dead, so she can have a fresh start. "What if she got square with the medical board, but PUH wouldn't hire her back? What if she, I don't know, took a job in some rural nowhere hospital where she could be a hero and not a pariah? What if she's *hoping* for someone to find her, so she can tell them to fuck off?"

As Maggie spoke, Jess leaned her body further and further and further away while Maggie relayed her theory, as if there were a stench that had attached itself to her body with this line of thinking. Maggie's hands were running through her hair as she spoke, loosening up the hold of her ponytail and causing various strands to stand straight up, making her head look like one of those plasma balls at Spencer Gifts.

"Why is this so important to you, Maggie? I just, I'm pretty sure she's dead," said Jess. "It was listed in the alumni magazine, you know."

SHE AIN'T DEAD MA'AM, Frank shouted at Jess, who refused to hear it. Maggie winced at Frank's volume in her ear.

Jess looked on Maggie's face with concern, or condescension, or disdain, depending on what filter you used to parse her face. The face a cop makes to a lost child at a carnival. The face a daughter makes to her demented mother who has forgotten her name. The face a toddler makes to a previously untried vegetable. Just as Maggie was about to launch into her next theory, her watch buzzed to pull her back to the present. A *p*Value* message, but it was from @dancindoctorjack, reminding her that the noon teaching session was starting.

"Damn, I gotta go." Maggie shut the browser abruptly and stood up, looking direct-to-camera with a wink before securing her workstation and rising out of her chair.

"Was that a *p*Value message?*" Jess followed behind Maggie toward the door.

Maggie reached up to remove the band from her ponytail, smoothed her hair back down into a more laminar order, and re-banded it. "It's a long story."

"Yeah, I guess so," said Jess, her face the way a tourist looks at a man holding a sign on the street corner. "You want to grab a drink later?"

"Yeah, sure, whatever," Maggie spat out before catching herself to correct her tone. "Yeah! I mean. Yes, for sure. Thanks, Jess. For listening to me."

Some people, Frank said, *just don't appreciate a good mystery when they see one.*

With that, Maggie left Jess behind in the lounge, as the doctors (and non-doctors who were close enough for the purposes of this lounge) lined up to receive their steam-table portion of Vegetable Lasagna and their side of Caesar salad. Lasagna that would feel in that moment as if it were free, because it wasn't paid for at the point of consumption. Lasagna that was not, in fact, free, because nothing was these days.

The hallways were now crowded with the lunchtime buzz, and Maggie zigged and zagged until she came to an elevator whose door was just opening as she walked by, inviting her to slip inside. She squeezed into a back corner as a group of medical students excitedly pushed into the car alongside her, trapping her with their frenetic energy and overstuffed backpacks. She was meant to be going up to the sixth floor, but after the doors closed she felt the drop in her stomach, signaling the car was actually going down. *Shit.* The only thing for it was to wait.

She distracted herself with $p*Value$ as the students jockeyed over mnemonics. *Some Lovers Try Positions That They Can't Handle* one student was saying to another, a statement that Maggie recognized as a stand-in for the carpal bones of the hand. *No no*, said another, *I prefer Scabby Lucy Tried Posting Hours after Copulating Two Twins.*

Jamie, 39, Fisheries Biologist. There may be a lot of fish in the sea, but I prefer fish in the river. Picture of her in fishing waders and nothing else, one overall hanging down provocatively like a 90s boy band member. Swipe left. The students continued. *So Long To Pinky Here Comes The Thumb. Oh, that's cute!*

Maggie looked up as the elevator gave a *ding* and a shudder as they arrived at the end point and the students filed out. *Level M*, it said. *M for. . .oh, right,* Maggie thought. She was hit with a wave of nostalgia and nausea as a familiar smell wafted through the doors. As the students filed out, she put her foot in front of the elevator door to keep it from closing, and leaned her head out into the hallway to take a peek. She could see a couple of the students doing Dr. Jack dance moves as they shimmied down the hallway, one coherent (Flatus? Nodule?) of hope and promise, walking so eagerly toward suffering.

She could warn them, but what good would it do? Had she the runway and the flux capacitor, could she go back in time to find her and Al and the rest of her class, skipping down these halls just like these excited students not long ago? Could she tell them, *quit medicine, travel the world, spend time with your family, now before they learn to hate you*? Now, in the present day, could she run after these students, yelling into the sky like a modern-day-Cassandra? *I do not see your beauty of old or hands warmed by burnt ships, but your lacerated limbs and those famous shoulders savaged by heavy chains,* she could say to them, as they laughed and laughed and laughed and said, *OK, Boomer.*

As she looked on, the students' feet lifted off the ground, and their bodies began to float up, up, up until they burst through the roof and into the mid-day sky, where a murder of benevolent crows swooped them up by their collars and carried them away to the nearby mountaintop. *You'll be safe there,* Maggie said to them, *trust me.*

Some Ladies Think People Have Come To Treason, the students yelled back from the mountain. Maggie was broken from her vision by Frank's voice.

I don't know what those motherfuckers were talkin' about, but I sure know a lost cause when I see one.

Maggie stepped back into the elevator and pushed the button for level six. On the way up, she was back into *p*Value,* swiping away a veterinarian in a bucket hat, a woman in a bowtie whose profession was listed as "PhDork," and a shirtless research scientist holding a guitar as if it were a baby. She felt the floor under her feet as the elevator lifted her own body up, up, up. The floor accelerated rapidly, until she herself was shot out the top of the elevator shaft and into the shroud of the city's cloud cover. She looked around at the apex for the crows to take her away, but found none.

Ding. The elevator opened, and Maggie headed back to the Green Team workroom.

Maggie arrived at the Green Team workroom at seven past the hour. Hearing through the door that the teaching session had already begun, she opened the door stealthily in that way you do to avoid disturbing the room, holding the handle of the door to prevent it from making a disruptive *clunk* that might draw eyeballs your way. She eyed a table of cafeteria pizza along the back wall and crept in that direction as quietly as she could with her heavy shoes. A nephrologist had everyone's attention at the white board on the other end of the room, having already drawn the haphazard curlicues of a massive nephron which was being labeled with various transporters and electrolytes with arrow-headed lines. The arrows had probably made sense at the time they were drawn, but looked for all the world now like the scrawling of a madman hell bent on launching positively charged missiles at a Flying Spaghetti Monster. At the back wall, Jack was leaning with his ankles crossed, thumb going mad with right-swiping, his free hand doing half-Vogue dance moves to an imagined beat. He gave Maggie a cursory head-nod, but kept at it.

Maggie folded a slice in one hand and put her attention to the board. The nephrologist was writing out drug names next to a squiggly line on the board, refusing to use brand names and thereby making the whole room wait while he spelled out *Empaglifolzin, Canagliflozin, Dapagliflozin* in sloppy and illegible cursive. Maggie relented and pulled out *p*Value*.

Jonathan, 47, Respiratory Tech. Taking breath control to the next level. Picture of him standing in front of a brick wall, holding a bouquet of flowers.

That guy? Frank interrupted her peaceful swiping. *That guy looks like a mark I once followed for an ex-wife. Turned out to be one of those fur-suit enthusiasts. Might be the same guy, now that I think of it. Got some great pictures, ex-wife was happy. She was a real looker, too.*

Maggie let loose an involuntary and too-loud sigh that brought Jack's gaze and raised eyebrows her way. She gave him a sheepish and apologetic wave and returned to her phone, giving Frank a *shutup-willyou* look as she did.

As she swiped left, the sound of a buzzing pager clattering on the table cut through the lecture, and Henry startled from what seemed like a waking nap to grab it and smash the buttons to quiet it. He stared at the message for a second, and then passed the pager over to Olive, who was cutting her slice of pizza up with a knife and fork delicately, while pausing to take notes in a bullet journal. Olive's eyes grew wide and she looked to the back of the room to find Maggie and summoned her to the table. What Maggie was shown when she shuffled quietly over was the result of Mr. Williams' CT scan, which she scrolled through, nodding to Olive with a somber face.

Told you so, said Frank, as he kicked his cowboy boots up onto the table and leaned back with satisfaction. *I gotta say, I told you so.*

Frank may have told her so, but it was something that Maggie already knew. Nice people die. Mean people live forever. Even in the face of this, it felt good to be right about it. Did that make her a mean person? Would that in turn extend her life?

Henry's pager went off again, just as he was starting to settle back into his lunch-time lean, and his eyes rolled along with a plosive sigh. He got up from the table, lifting his chair off the floor slightly as he pushed it back to avoid the gnawing squeak that a chair moving over an over-waxed floor would give, and tip-toed over to Jack, who only barely looked up from his swiping but acknowledged Henry's presence with a soft, *mmhmm?*

"New admission in the ER, should I see them now or wait 'til they hit the floor?" Henry said. *Hit the floor* in the hospital means your patient has arrived at their assigned bed, though it sounds like your patient is stumbling drunk. Jack rolled his eyes up briefly without raising his head and, without saying a word, simply waved his hand over toward the door. Jack then looked over at Maggie, and gave a similar gesture to her, waving to Maggie, to Henry, to the door, to Maggie again mouthing *go go go go* as if they were rolling out on a clandestine mission. On her way out the door, Maggie's watch buzzed with a new message from *p*Value.*

From @dancingdoctorjack:

Thought this would be a good case for a noob, you'll see.

Maggie, walking silently behind an annoyed Henry, took out her phone and responded back:

From @magneatomd

You misspelled 'expert'

FYI, fever guy has colon cancer with mets.

What's my prize?

Maggie sent that with a smile.

BOO-YA, IN YOUR FACE, motherfucker, said Frank. Maggie felt the rush of her brain's reward system cashing out into her ego bank, *ka-ching.* Maggie did not build this system; rather she was built by it. The system is a Vegas slot machine into which you are feeding your life savings, designed to hit a big win just before you spend your last dollar. You know you shouldn't keep going, but you do anyway, because the high is worth it, and because this is the system. The system knows a light is needed at the end of the tunnel, and even though the light is a dumpster fire, the warmth on your face feels great.

Maggie put her phone away and caught up to Henry waiting at the elevator, scrolling through the new admission's patient record on an iPad with his glasses flipped up to the top of his head.

"Looks like an arson lung patient," he said. "We've gotten a lot this week."

"Arson lung?" This wasn't a condition Maggie had heard of previously, and wondered if it was slang for something.

"Almost all young people, too. Kinda sad. Mostly we just babysit them and titrate oxygen and nebs until it clears up. You don't actually have to come if you don't want to, it's not that interesting."

"I'm sure I'll learn something," said Maggie, hoping to not seem like a total idiot on her first day. The elevator gave a *ding* and the doors opened, and Henry and Maggie found themselves a lucky early-afternoon elevator to themselves. Henry used the opportunity to give Maggie a running commentary from the patient's ER notes.

"Looks like a John Doe — lots of these arson lung patients are. They don't tell us their names and don't bring their ID so we can't tell the cops, or something, I dunno. Sometimes we recognize 'em, it'll be the same frequent flyer for a while and then they stop coming, we assume they got arrested."

The elevator shuddered as it took off downward, and Maggie's hand gripped the side rail while trying to look calm and collected, like an attending should.

"Why would they get arrested? Not sure I follow."

"They're fire chasers. They hunt for Burning Man to try and catch him, or join him, or post on KnockKnock or something. That's how they get arson lung; it's just a smoke inhalation injury is all it is. Cops keep catching 'em thinking they *are* Burning Man, but who knows. Fires just keep going."

Of course, Burning Man. Maggie thought about the box of letters she'd tried to will to the Burning Man, wondering if there was a way she could summon him again with Al's mail.

"What do you think? About Burning Man, I mean. Do you think it's these kids?" Maggie's watch buzzed, and she pulled the sleeve of her white coat down to cover it.

"Who knows, man. Ain't my job to figure it out. I just treat 'em and street 'em." Henry was busy entering admission orders as quickly as he could muster into his tablet, most of the orders suggested by MaX. Chime, chime, chime, said MaX as Henry accepted its suggestions, and the chimes made them both feel good for reasons they couldn't explain.

"You know what, Henry? Why don't you let me talk to this one. It sounds like you've seen this a million times and I've never seen it yet since I'm new in town. I'll even write the note."

Henry looked up in surprise. "Really?"

"Yeah, really. You deserve a break."

The elevator spat them out into the Emergency Room lobby, which in the mid-day held only a smattering of minor injuries and anxious parents. A young couple holding an inconsolable newborn who would be told later *it's just colic.* A middle-aged woman in a wheelchair with an ice-packed ankle. A masked older person in a corner coughing and coughing and coughing and coughing. Maggie and Henry held their breath as they walked past this person and badged through the door into the department, which was a winding maze of sliding-door cubicles that extended to fill nearly the entire ground floor. In spite of the sleepy quietude of the waiting room, the back hallways were a study in pure chaos — moaning coming from *somewhere* that no one seemed concerned by, an elder voice periodically yelling *hello hello is anyone there*, a screaming toddler, nurses in sturdy sneakers wearing down the floor wax with quick steps that left subtle lines connecting all the rooms to the computer workstations in the middle. Henry led the way to a back corner, to the room where John Doe was being stowed.

The sliding glass door was closed tightly, and on the other side a curtain had been pulled, and Maggie could see the lights were off in the room. Maggie gave the door an assertive knock, then cracked it just a bit, saying at the same time "Knock-knock! Doctor's here!"

She paused for a moment, as if to allow for an objection or a gathering of whatever might need gathering, and, hearing nothing, opened the door and curtain wide enough to let in the light from the hallway. This was a little routine she did every time she entered a room in the hospital, day or night (save emergencies), and had done for as long as she could remember. This redundant pre-entry warning system had been learned from the doctors who trained her, who learned from the doctors before them, who learned from the doctors before them, and so on and so on, a lineage that reached back to the very first doctor to inadvertently walk in on a patient masturbating in whatever passed for a hospital, and who had been so scarred as to pass on that trauma for a dozen generations. After she gave her pupils time to adjust to the dim light, Maggie knocked again, and walked a few steps into the room.

What she saw atop the bed was a body covered all-the-way-over by crisp white hospital sheets and curled into a tight ball, giving it the look of a melting ice cream scoop atop the undulating platform of the pressure-relieving hospital air mattress. Within this forbidden confection, periodic and paroxysmal cough-heaves gave away the patient's position and affliction both. A long cannula lay tangled and abandoned by the bedside, spewing concentrated oxygen into the general milieu while carbon dioxide no doubt built up within the blanket-cave.

Maggie knocked again, this time on the inside of the door. "Knock-knock," she said a bit louder, "Doctor's here." The cover's edge was then pulled tighter underneath the sleeping form, a reflex that Maggie thought might suggest that this John Doe still lives with his parents. "John? It's Doctor Owens, I'm going to be taking care of you upstairs. We need to talk for a minute."

Insisting vehemently that a sleeping person wake up to talk to you is a behavior reserved for a select group of people. Mothers with children running late for school. Prison guards. Spurned lovers. Doctors. Cops clearing the park benches. Common courtesy is a luxury these people have none of. You don't go to the hospital to get rest, you go to the hospital to get well. You think you can sleep when you're dead? Hell no, we don't even let the dead sleep in the hospital. We punch them in the chest until they can wake up and give us the goddamn family history that our attending asked for.

Maggie took a few warning steps toward the bed, audible-on-purpose in her clunky Danskos, to give the young man a chance to realize they weren't going away. The covers were still clutched around the head like armor. Cough. Cough. A muffled voice spoke out. "Can you come back later?"

"It's the doctor." Maggie said this as if it were explanation enough.

"Can you come back later, Doctor?"

"Sorry, buddy, we've got to see you now. You're being admitted to the hospital. We'll let you go back to sleep in a minute. We have to make a plan for your care," Maggie says, cruelly turning on the bright overhead light to make it clear that she meant business. We are all capable of inhumane behavior, if given the right motivation and an understanding that it is for the greater good. This is a lesson humanity learns over and over and over again. Maggie is not the system, but the system is working through her, and the system gets what it wants.

A tuft of cropped blue hair appeared from under the cover, then slowly the form of a human emerged. Within two squinting eyelids, two pastel blue eyes peeked out, pointing directly at Maggie with post-sleep eye-daggers. Cough. Cough.

"Here I am, I'm alive, okay? Now can I sleep?"

"I'm your doctor for today, Dr. Owens."

As Maggie's eyes locked with these pastel eyes she stopped in realization, furrowed her brow, and tilted her head to the side. "Ja—" she started to say, until the blue-haired and blue-eyed person abruptly cut her off with a coughing fit that sprayed a fine gray mist onto the white hospital sheet in front of them. They were shaking their head furiously and holding a hand up in a *stop* formation. Maggie took the meaning, looking over at Henry, who was swiping around his tablet, not seeming to be paying attention. She mouthed, silently this time, *Jax?*

I thought you said you weren't a nurse, mouthed Jax back at her, a sentiment Maggie luckily could not quite parse. Maggie looked again over at Henry, who seemed to be reviewing lab results on the tablet.

"Hey, Henry? Can you do me a favor and find a nurse to bring in some more nebulizer solution? Looks like we're running on empty here." She reached over and turned off the wall valve that had been feeding the errant line, and the room fell silent. Henry nodded, tucking the tablet into the back of his scrub pants and ducking through the curtain. Maggie shut the sliding door all the way as he left, and then took a seat on the rolling stool and slid it up to the side of Jax's bed.

"So," said Maggie. "What do *you* think about all those fires?"

Jax blushed.

"You mean the ones" — cough — "in the Amazon? Never" — cough — "heard of 'em."

Oh, this motherfucker thinks he's clever, Frank grumbled from the corner, *Don't let him off the hook so easily.* Maggie was nodding, slowly, with just enough of a smile on her face to disarm Jax, but not enough to look goofy.

"I thought you said you weren't a nurse," Jax said.

"Not a nurse, just a doctor."

"Ohhhhhh, I'm sorry."

"Don't apologize, please. Don't. Nurses are great. I'm just not one of 'em."

No shit, you're a DOCTOR? Frank said with surprise from the corner. *Guess they'll let broads do any fuckin' thing these days!* Maggie's fingers gripped her thigh to prevent her face from grimacing.

"So," she continued, "what *were* you doing in the alley last night?"

That's right! Frank egged her on from the corner. *Don't believe the official story! Not for a second!*

Jax was looking down at their hands, which Maggie now noticed were not the smooth and thin hands of an IT keyboard-jockey, but were worn, ruddy, with red burn marks on several fingertips and rough calluses partially ripped off of the palms. Jax continued to look down, smiling quietly and tucking their hands under the black-splattered hospital blanket. "Are you gonna tell on me?"

"What?"

"Are you like, required to tell them who I am?" Jax had a look of desperation on their face that they were trying to hide with a sly smile. Their eyes gave it away, though.

You've got him cornered, Maggie! Cornered! Frank was shadow boxing with what remained of his hands, his phalanges and severed tendons flopping around like pompoms. *Get the cuffs!*

"No, of course not. I'm your doctor, not a detective. Your secrets are safe with me."

Gahhd dammit, I hate this good cop shit. You gotta go in for the kill! Frank's shredded boxing-hands looked so ridiculous that it was taking all of Maggie's effort not to crack up.

"Alright, alright" — cough — "alright." Jax caved too easily, like they'd been waiting to be outed. "Alright. I *might* have been out looking at fires last night. Our conversation got us curious, you know? It was my first time doing it though, I *swear.*" Maggie tried to parse their face for signs of a lie. Eyes darting up to the left, increased blink rate, fidgeting hands, things she'd learned on late night police procedural TV. Jax was working hard to breathe, tensing their abdominal muscles to push air out to make room for each next breath. Jax held their side with both hands to brace the ribs as they went in for another round of coughing. Maggie waited for a break before she continued.

"First time, huh? I mean, that cough isn't any first time cough. That cough is a *habit.*"

This was an interviewing technique that doctors had borrowed from detective procedurals and prison informants. State it as a fact, like the evidence is already in the evidence locker and you better come clean or risk losing your plea deal. Jax didn't bite, they just kept coughing. Maggie tried a different spin.

"It's not anything to me, you understand. I'm just here to take care of you. As a *doctor.*" She took a quick and pointed peek back at

Frank when she said the word *doctor*. "I'm sworn to confidentiality, right? I'm on your side. But you should know that some of the old downtown buildings have asbestos insulation, lead paint, those types of things. Not to mention fiberglass and volatile printer ink and all that stuff can get into your lungs if it's caught up in the smoke. You know how those Ground Zero workers after 9/11 had all those lung problems? Some of them died from it. So it *really* would help me to know how long you've been doing this."

This might have been true on some level that Maggie needed this medical information. But in her heart of hearts, this was not why she asked. Jax laughed, a laugh that was punctuated by a few uncovered hacks and then followed by a deep and effortful breath.

"You know I was born *after* 9/11."

Maggie didn't respond, she just nodded, leaving a silence between them that extended beyond the point of awkwardness, another interrogation technique doctors shared amongst themselves, a long and awkward silence being to most people a form of quiet torture in line with waterboarding. If you stop talking for long enough, people will just tell you things to make it stop. Maggie made the most empty-vessel face that she could and kept her breath quiet. Jax squirmed in the bed.

Like your style, Owens, said Frank from the corner. *This dude's gonna crack.*

"I met 'em, you know," Jax said.

Maggie put on the stone face that she used for occasions when patients revealed shocking information, a face she had copied from Barbara Walters' interview with Mary Kay Letourneau. A face that said oh-how-interesting, but at a distance. A face careful not to offer approval, but also not saying *what-the-fuck.*

"Hmm," said Maggie softly, barely audible, a voice you had to lean in to hear. Frank was right, Jax had the look of an overfull water balloon, just a slight jiggle away from bursting. Maggie said nothing, and they continued.

"Burning Man? Well, we say Burning Person because we don't want to assume. I saw them. At least, I *think* so. The fires have got a pattern, you know? Where they show up. The kinds of stuff they like to go after. It's just one person, though. The same one over and over. I don't care what the cops say."

Maggie kept nodding, nodding, leaving space for more. Face like an empty canvas. Eyes like a void. Jax continued.

"You know we can kinda predict where the fires will hit? Been able to for a coupla weeks." Jax was giving up more than they'd intended to. Maggie was practically invisible, the information passing right through her, and Jax continued. "We go where the pattern leads us, we wait, and sure enough." Maggie's watch buzzed to let her know she was holding her breath, but she paid it no mind.

"So," she said in her smallest, meekest, tiniest but most urgent voice, "you saw them?"

"Yeah. I hid behind a dumpster and saw their shoes. Chuck Taylors, but with a pattern on 'em."

Maggie didn't dare say a word. She just nodded and waited. Jax went on.

"Arsonists always come back, you know. That's a known thing about arsonists: they have to see their work. So we've been staying behind, hiding in the smoke, looking for those shoes. We find them in the crowd and stand nearby."

"Did you say anything?" Maggie had fully departed from medical intent, and was venturing into a space in her brain that was occupied by a childhood Harriet the Spy obsession. "Did you get their name?"

Was it Alice, by any chance? Maggie's mind was desperately trying to pull every thread together all at once. *Did she have a face that was all of everything altogether? Could you not take your eyes off of her even if you wanted to?*

"Not yet. I'm working up the nerve to talk to 'em." Jax looked right at Maggie now, making eye contact for the first time in a minute. "We followed them, though. They sleep in a blue hammock on the hillside, just down there. Super high up in the trees."

"Are you sure it was the real Burning Man? Or, Burning Person?"

Jax shrugged. "I mean, I'm pretty sure. But, whatever. I guess time will tell, right?"

"Yeah, time will tell."

Maggie ruminated on that. People said that a lot, that time would tell. But in reality, time was pretty good at keeping secrets, washing away the fingerprint oils and eroding the fine details and paving over the footprints and burning up the available textile evidence. DNA breaks down, data corrupts, photographs fade. History belongs to the present, time splitting the universe as it skips along the surface of space. The dinosaurs had feathers or scales, the *T. Rex* was a vicious killer or a kind scavenger, what did it matter when eventually everything would be covered over with slime mold emboldened by rising sea levels. Time, eventually, will keep all secrets. But the Burning Person, Maggie supposed, could still be known, and the possibility of that identity being revealed was thrilling.

Jax coughed a little more and held their side with one hand. "Shoot, hurts to cough so bad," they said, looking sheepishly over at Maggie. "Do you think I could get, like, an oxy or something? Not a lot! Just like, one? Maybe two?"

Jax asked this question with a shrinking reserve, the way a person asks when they know the answer is likely to be inversely correlated with how urgently they seem to want it. This phrasing confirmed it must not be Jax's first time in a hospital, because people in pain have to learn to have this dance with the keepers of pain medicine. There are no winners in this dance-battle, because the doctors who say yes every time are basically drug dealers and the doctors who say no every time are definitely sociopaths, and somewhere between these extremes people assume there will be a balance of yes and no that allows someone to be a human being, but there isn't. There are just individual moments judged on this binary, as all doctors oscillate between dual states of pushover and sadist every time the question comes up.

"Yeah," Maggie said, putting her palms up in front of her body as if to demonstrate a lack of weapons. "Yeah, of course." Maggie walked over to the workstation to oblige, having chosen her side in this battle long ago. She typed o-x-y- into an order field, and MaX helpfully completed her thought with the dosing and frequency and she signed it and got the chime. MaX, it seemed, had also chosen a side, a side that aligned with satisfied patients and Press Ganey scores and Sackler family trust funds, and also on occasion with compassion and ease. "Nurse should be in soon with it."

"Wait, aren't you the, oh, never mind," Jax started to say as Henry arrived back to the room, holding a bucket full of tubing and plastic twist-off vials full of nebulizer juice.

"Hey, hey, sorry I took so long. I couldn't find a nurse so, I don't know, I think this is all the right stuff." With her back to Henry, Maggie mimed to Jax that she was zipping her lips shut, the universal sign of a kept secret.

"Henry, do you know how to set it up?"

Henry shook his head no, shrugging his shoulders comically like a dad in a commercial for laundry detergent.

"Alright then, let's teach you a useful skill, shall we?" Maggie snaked the tubing from the wall and over to Jax's bedside, showing Henry how to connect the plastic end piece to the tubing, fill the chamber with liquid, and turn the wall valve all the way up. The pipe hissed with vaporous output and Maggie handed it to Jax.

"There you go," Maggie said, handing the steaming kazoo over to a still-coughing Jax, "since you like to inhale smoke so much." She winked at them as she said this, like a cool teacher might. She then gathered up the waste packaging into a makeshift bindle with a blue underpad that had been cast onto the floor, little bits of plastic and wrappers, and the spent container from the last treatment. She tossed it all into a large red bin in the room that would eventually offload its cargo to somewhere else that Maggie tried not to think about, maybe directly to an underground landfill, maybe shot into space, who knows.

"We'll check on you later," Maggie said as she and Henry stepped out and slid the door shut behind them.

After they were in the hall, Maggie stopped, looked at her watch, and looked over at Henry, who was typing away on his tablet. "Don't worry about the note. I already took care of it," he said. "Well, me and MaX. Should we head back to the workroom?"

"How about a break instead?"

Henry blinked, and blinked again. "Break?"

Maggie opened up her white coat pocket and gestured to the contents. Henry's eyes widened and he expelled his breath in percussive relief. "Oh, snap!"

"I smelled your vape earlier. Have you been out to the clearing before?"

Henry eyed his pager, then placed a hand on it as if it were a loaded gun in a holster that may be drawn at any second. "Are you sure?"

"You deserve it," said Maggie. "Probably. I know I do." Maggie was already leading them down the stairwell that led to the clearing, hand in pocket, finger slipped under the cover of her cigarette box, touching just the rough edge of the filter tip. "No one will die if we take a break, Henry."

Maggie was not the system. Henry was not the system. They could make non-system choices. They could head to the clearing for a smoke, like human beings. When they got to the clearing, they could stand in silence, thinking their separate thoughts while they inhaled their separate nicotines in near-unison in their separate nearby universes. They could stand there, in the middle of their work day, contemplating how the sun's rays bounce around in chaotic vectors through the tree leaves, making the afternoon sky look like stars above them. They could gaze off the hillside into the far distance across the waterfront, where a half-finished condo building had burned to the ground overnight and was still spewing some combination of steam and ash into a haze, and they could think of this as a type of very expensive ephemeral performance art, more beautiful for its impermanence. They could pointedly *not* run through their patient list, *not* use the tablet to place orders, *not* make a call to the nurse on the 7th floor who paged sixteen minutes ago asking if there were any new orders for a blood pressure reading of 147/76, *not* put in the potassium repletion for the patient on the 8th floor whose nurse just informed them of some leg cramps, and definitely, definitely *not* track down the med student to send him home.

Those things could lay in stasis for just one moment, time enough for these two people to do this small act of self-immolation that was just for them. Because they were not the system. And the system could only work through them if they were working. And they were on a break.

"Can I, um, ask you a question," said Henry, his face enveloped in a cloud of pleasant vanilla vapor, like a genie.

"Sure," said Maggie. She thinks he will be asking her for some kind of sage, attending-advice, something like *how do you achieve work-life balance* or *how do I calculate the total body water again* or *what is the name of that thing that happens to potassium in ketoacidosis.* She tried to steel her best adult face.

"Do you, like, microdose at all?" Henry was now holding out a small tincture bottle labeled *Happy Shit.*

"Microdose?" Maggie knew the term, but it had never been presented so directly to her before. "Like, mushrooms?" Maggie was doing her Barbara Walters face.

"Psilocybin," Henry said. "It's an extract now. *Legal,* you know. In case you were wondering."

"No," Maggie said. "I don't. I mean, I haven't. What's it like?"

"You should try it. It's like, everything just seems a little brighter. Almost all the residents are doing it. Better than a dumb SSRI or something."

"Hm," Maggie said. "I guess whatever helps, right?"

"Wanna try it?"

Henry suspended the dropper above his mouth, letting two drops fall on his tongue. He pinched the dropper between two fingers and offered it to Maggie, as if it were a joint.

Something tells me you don't need that shit to separate you from reality, says Frank, right as always.

"Not today," she said, "but thank you for thinking of me."

Maggie was almost down to the filter when her watch buzzed. She made the reflexive mistake of swiping at it, and found a message from DoCTR Debbie, letting her know that she needed to *stop by and get that form signed!!!* Near-simultaneously, Henry's pager went off, startling him and causing him to stuff his tincture bottle into his white coat pocket as if the pager would rat him out.

"Damn," he said, looking at the pager. "Nurse for the fever guy wants someone to go talk to him about his results."

"Maybe Dancin' Doctor Jack can do a sad tango to break the news," Maggie said, tossing her butt into the coffee can as she followed

Henry back toward the door, reaching in her pocket for the hand-sanitizer and the Altoid mint and the bathroom spray.

"You head back to the workroom," she told Henry as they started climbing the stairs. "I'm gonna make a stop back in the ER. I have a question I forgot to ask." Henry was already ten paces ahead of her on the stairs, pager going off again to call the 7th floor nurse about the elevated blood pressure, which was now 152/84, and *still without orders, please acknowledge.* He gave a thumbs-up sign back at her and continued to bound up, two at a time, because that was how all young and fit male residents took the stairs, as if they were firefighters making their way up a burning building to rescue a trapped grand-mother. Maggie didn't bound, but she did step more briskly up the stairs than she typically would, propelled by her idea.

A few minutes later she was standing outside Jax's room, taking a deep breath, a literal threshold in front of her. She raised a hand and rapped on the glass door.

"Knock-knock, it's Doctor Owens again." She slid the door just open, but left the curtain pulled. "Knock-knock?" She paused and heard no objection. She pulled the curtain just enough to peek her head through and found Jax awake and pointing a phone camera at her this time. They were breathing a bit easier after the nebulizer treat-ment, and now appeared to be live-streaming.

"Say hi to the people, Doctor. What do you have to say about American health care?" As Jax's halogen phone-light was cast into Maggie's eyes, she was briefly blinded and disoriented. She shielded her eyes like a celebrity might when faced with unwanted paparazzi, and froze for a minute, stammering.

"We're people, too," said Maggie. "Except the ones who are robots." She gestured to the workstation. "But I guess you'd probably know about that, wouldn't you, *John Doe?*"

Jax laughed, and the light from the phone shut off as they set it on their lap. "Thanks for the pain meds, doc. I already feel a *lot* better. You should try 'em sometime. They ever let you try 'em? They should let you try 'em." The medicine was not the system, but the system worked through it, giving it breath as it had for a hundred years. The medicine was not opium, but it wasn't *not* opium, either.

Maggie took a step inside the room, pulling the curtain behind her.

"Jax, you said you're good at finding people, right?" Jax nodded. "Do you. . .think you could help me find someone?" Maggie's face said both *no pressure* and *please, please, please.*

"Yeah, of course," said Jax. "Of course." There was a pause. "Um, I do still have a little pain. Do you think. . .you know. . ." Maggie cut them off by putting a finger to her lips. She nodded.

"Yeah, yeah. Whatever you need." It would be better if the question weren't fully asked. "I mean, I'll take care of you no matter if you help me or not, of course. Just so you know."

"Great." Jax was rubbing their hands together as if to start a small fire, and they pulled a beat-up MacBook covered in bumper stickers from under the bed covers. "Now tell me who you're lookin' for."

Maggie grabbed the rolling stool, and rolled up to the bedside and pulled the beat-up letter out of her pocket.

"Her name is Alice Power."

CHAPTER 10

PGY8

It was that blissful final month before the start of the pandemic, when stateside doctors had just *just* started to hear talk of the virus bantered about, but mostly as a kind of joke they would make any time a patient had a fever that was unexplained or arrived at the hospital with any history of recent travel. It was a time when everyone was still taking public transit and going to bars and concerts and sitting in lecture halls while neighbors coughed nearby and they were thinking nothing of it. They were not even hoarding toilet paper or surgical masks or concocting home hand-sanitizer recipes out of Everclear and vanilla extract. They were not even washing their hands after touching a doorknob, let alone wearing surgical masks to the grocery store or allowing six feet of social separation. They were not yet fashioning home-made air filters out of vacuum bags and Flex-Tape. No, they were just making jokes about pangolins and remembering how easily it seemed the *Ebola* virus had been defeated a few years earlier and thinking that it would be like that. They were bemoaning the inevitable institution of travel screening questions at hospital entry points, questions that would no doubt be more annoying than helpful until this all blew over. They were throwing away gloves after only a single use, as if they were *garbage.*

It had been an unusually cold February that year by West Coast standards, such that even the Midwest-hardened Maggie remembered it as colder than she expected, the grid of condo buildings seeming to funnel the wind into torpedo-tubes of cutting air that caught her by surprise as she walked to her destination on the waterfront. She could feel the shocked pink of her cheeks as she walked, hoping it would make her seem rosy and not clownish.

The bar Al had chosen was windowless, dim, and situated a few blocks past the far end of the strip of hospital-worker condos, in a part of the neighborhood that hadn't yet been caught up in the hospital-money net. The bar was mostly empty, and Maggie immediately spotted Al in the back. Al was meticulously racking up balls at a far corner pool table, lifting and spinning the balls into position with a level of practiced perfection that was wholly unnecessary for the setting. She would thrust the rack forward and back and forward again, shake her head, spin some balls individually, and then thrust the rack into position again. Maggie almost didn't recognize her, as she had shaved her head to the skin in the time since Maggie last saw her, and the hanging pool-table light was reflecting a green hue off of a now-reflective dome that made her seem downright alien. *Rack. Re-rack. Rack again.* Maggie leaned against the bar, watching Al work but catching the attention of the bartender in her peripheral vision.

"Scotch and Soda," Maggie said to this faceless person, "with a twist of lime." Al was running a hand over her head in circles, as if it were the belly of a buddha, and hadn't yet noticed Maggie's arrival. After a moment of intent staring, a loud snap next to Maggie's ear brought her attention to the bartender beside her.

"Eight dollars," he or she said, as a scotch and soda appeared in Maggie's hand. Maggie threw a ten down, still not looking at the man-or-whatever.

Maggie didn't like Scotch, and she didn't like soda, and her acid reflux would rebel against the addition of lime, but she liked the aesthetic of this drink in this moment, in this bar, in this situation. She was here, after all. She was using her allotted Continuing Medical

Education travel stipend to spend a week in a board exam review course at a downtown hotel conference room, a time and a date and a location she has chosen for this review course for the outwardly stated reasons that it did not conflict with spring break hospital coverage and *actually I've been meaning to try and catch up with everyone*, and *I hear that review course is top notch* and Christopher had outwardly accepted these reasons. Maggie had never failed a test in her life, and a full week of board review was certainly overkill, and to fly across the country for such a thing was more than unnecessary, but Maggie seemed set on it. Certainly wouldn't have anything to do with Al, whose name still popped up occasionally on the screen of Maggie's phone with text-pictures of various triangles and erupting volcanoes and fecal references and other in-jokes that Christopher was tangentially aware of.

Do you think you'll catch up with Alice while you're there, Christopher had dropped casually while washing the dishes as Maggie sat at the table working a Sudoku.

Oh, I dunno, I kinda doubt it, Maggie had said, less than one day after sending Al a text to say she's coming to town and suggesting a drink. *I'll probably just buckle down in my hotel room with the question bank and a glass of wine,* she had said to Christopher, having then spent the day checking her phone every two to three minutes for a response.

And Al did respond, didn't she, and here they were. Maggie leaned against the bar, trying to look casual while wearing a low-cut blouse underneath a leather jacket, and eye makeup for the first time in five years. Maggie held her hardened scotch and soda in one hand, her other thumb hooked over a belt loop in a pose she thought might make her look casual and cool. In this repose, she sidled up to Al, who continued to thrust billiard balls into near-perfect position on the table, over and over and over, reluctant to call it good. Al was wearing a loose and unbuttoned flannel shirt over a faded *Mudhoney* T-Shirt, circa Portland 1997, and that combined with her now-bald head completed a grunge rock look that was unfamiliar to Maggie.

"Howdy pard'ner," Al said to Maggie with a grin as she came into focus, looking her up and down exaggeratedly for her amusement. "You new 'round these parts?"

Maggie laughed and set her drink down on the edge of the pool table, opening her arms to give Al a hug. Al obliged with a brief embrace that ended in the confusing combined body language of a hearty pat on the back followed by a lingering hand on Maggie's arm as Al moved away and back to the table.

Al positioned her hands over the rack again, and Maggie noticed a fine tremor as Al lifted the plastic triangle again, a vibration that knocked the balls just enough to send them drifting apart. Al's lips curled inward in frustration as she stared down at the table. "I'm going to get another drink," she said, giving Maggie a wink.

Maggie watched Al walk away to the bar, noting her pants riding low and loose on her hips, a style choice or a consequence of weight loss, or both. Al stood at the bar chatting with the bartender, taking a shot first and then waiting for the bartender to make another drink. Maggie, always impulsively useful, set to arranging the balls back in their triangular home, and lifted the plastic stay just as Al returned with a drink in hand.

"Nice rack," Al said, except she was looking directly at Maggie and not the table, and dropping her eyes *just so*. Maggie dropped her head to the side to give Al the *you-stinker* look that was so well worn from their lab days, but the corners of her mouth gave away an underlying feeling that was not exactly exasperation.

"Thanks," said Maggie. "All that hormone-laden midwestern cheese has its benefits." As Maggie said this, she cheekily put a hand on one boob and gave it a little bounce before she could stop herself.

"No wonder Christopher doesn't want to leave Missouri, I guess," Al remarked with a wink.

"Oh, Christopher is lobbying to ban hormones in farm animals, you know. So I doubt he's probably noticed. For what it's worth."

"Oh, is he now? Saint Christopher's goodness knows no bounds, I suppose." Al was lining her cue up on the cue ball, eyes laser focused now on the task at hand. Maggie leaned against the table from the other end, hair long and loose over her shoulders, drink in hand, dripping condensation onto her fingers.

"No comment."

Al broke with a casual confidence that suggested she was practiced, somehow exerting only a tiny amount of effort to produce an unusual vector of force, like there was some hidden impulse on the tip of her cue that had amplified her motion. Three balls sunk into pockets as she looked down her nose at the table and moved to call her next shot.

"No comment, huh? Things going that well in Missour-uh?" She pronounced the state name with an only slight exaggeration of its signature accent. "Is that all you have to say about that?" Maggie shook her head.

Al pointed her cue at the corner pocket, saying, "Nine ball," before sending said ball into the corner pocket. Maggie took a drink of her scotch, and set the drink on the edge of the table to adjust her skin-tight jacket, which was quickly becoming uncomfortable. She regretted the choice of leather now, and considered taking it off, but felt she still needed the armor of it. She settled on pulling down the sleeves and giving her shoulders a little shimmy to break the seal that the impenetrable fabric had made on her sweaty skin. Al wasn't looking at her, having moved on to her next shot, eleven ball, side pocket.

"Is it just me, or did your hands get steadier after you got that extra drink?" Maggie asked, a question that was standing in for another question Maggie was afraid to ask. *Differential diagnosis,* she would have written if this were a patient note, *alcohol withdrawal, generalized anxiety disorder, essential tremor, thyroid disease, early-onset Parkinson's.*

"You know Maggie," Al said pointedly, "you don't always have to be so goddamn *smart.* You could turn it off if you wanted to." Al was looking Maggie right in the eyes, icebergs piercing right into the earthen brown of Maggie's own eyes. Maggie said nothing in return, leaving the silence to sit between them, a vacuum waiting for words to give it air. An internist knows this game in a way a surgeon never will, and Al was the first to break.

"Benign Essential Tremor," said Al. "I've had it since med school."

Benign Essential Tremor was almost certainly named by someone who didn't themselves suffer from the condition, which sends its sufferers hands into oscillating harmonic patterns that frustrate normal activities like holding a glass of water, writing in cursive, or lifting a pool rack off the table smoothly. Though Benign Essential Tremor has a number of potential medical treatments, many patients discover on their own that alcohol can smooth out the edges of the tremor without the need for medical intervention.

"Al," said Maggie. She sat on the precipice of saying the next thing on her mind, which was *but you're a surgeon.* Maggie thought back to the cadaver lab, the flask of tequila that Al had tucked away in her pocket, the shaking hand she had seen from time to time that she'd taken for nervousness or caffeine overload. *But you're a surgeon,* Maggie thought again, loud enough that she felt certain Al could hear it.

"Don't worry about me," Al said, returning her attention back to the pool table as a means to end this line of questioning. "I manage it." Al smoothly put a hand on the table, positioned her cue with stone-cold precision atop her index finger, and sent the nine ball into a side pocket. "See? Steady as she goes."

Maggie nodded and changed the subject. "You know I had my five-year anniversary at Jackson County Memorial this year," Maggie said as she watched Al circling the table to hunt her next shot. "Christopher and I both did. You know we've been there longer than anyone else in the department."

"Oh boy, I hope they gave you some kind of special plaque to hang on your wall." Al sent the thirteen and fifteen careening in opposite directions, with a chaotic energy that surely couldn't have been purposeful, except that it was, and both balls disappeared below the table with a fricative subterranean roll, back to the ball return.

"I got a T-shirt, actually."

"NO!" Alice stood straight up and pointed the pool cue right at Maggie as she said this.

"Oh, yes. An actual T-shirt."

"What did it say?"

"Oh, it was personalized with my name on the back, like a sports jersey. And it had a big number 5, and underneath that it said: 'Team Player.'"

"Oh *boy.* Personalized! You must have felt so special."

"I also got a coupon for one free coffee in the cafeteria."

"Hot diggity dog."

Al finally missed a shot, (on purpose, perhaps) and handed the cue over to Maggie. Maggie walked around the table to survey her options. She decided to try for the six ball, which was stopped just shy of a side pocket. As she leaned over to take her shot, she found herself consciously squeezing her shoulders together in that way that would pump up her cleavage just slightly. *Do women even like this kind of thing?* She looked up at Al for a second, who was looking down at her with a smile. Maggie looked away again and took her shot. The cue ball managed to miss the six entirely, shooting itself straight into the side pocket and rolling to the ball return.

"Ah, well. That's my luck. Did you know Christopher's the Chief of Medicine now?"

Al laughed for a moment and then stopped laughing as she realized it wasn't a joke.

"At a hospital where *you* work?"

Maggie nodded. "Yep. After he was promoted, one of the admin leaders actually *congratulated* me. Wouldn't I be proud to have kids with the Chief of Medicine, she said. She wasn't joking."

"Every girl's dream, to be honest." Al took her next shot, missing badly, and handed the pool cue back to Maggie, who set her drink on the table and leaned over again to take a shot, this time looking Al directly in the eye while she did it.

"You can tell me you told me so if you want," Maggie said.

"That's not my style," said Al. "Though I think I did."

"NO DRINKS ON POOL TABLES," came a booming voice from behind the bar, and Maggie startled and stood up, picking her drink off the table and giving an apologetic glance back at the bar.

"Sorry!" she said loud enough for the bartender to hear. *"Must be an East Coast guy,"* she followed as an aside for just Al.

"Yep, that's why I like this place. None of this west coast passive subtext bullshit. It's refreshing."

"Huh. I see." Maggie paused, holding one hand akimbo on her hip, tilting her head in that way that a woman does. She had taken this stance with Alice before, long ago, and it hadn't worked then, but who's keeping score. "Well, do you have anything refreshing to say?"

"Not in the slightest. But do you want to see my place? It's just down the street in the Daniel building."

Maggie paused, taking a deep breath and looking away as if the question had been written on a far wall. She let the breath out and nodded. She crossed her arms in front of her chest, squeezing them again for emphasis.

"Yeah, yeah, of course I want to see your place."

Al hung her cue back on the wall, leaving the game unfinished, and grabbed her own coat off the nearby stool. She gestured for Maggie to follow her out, which Maggie did after draining the last bit of her drink, cringing as it hit her stomach, but also wishing there were more of it.

There would be more drinks that night, but not much more conversation. Al's hands, Maggie would have occasion to discover, were strong, and skilled, and smooth when they needed to be, as if proving a point.

The next morning, the two sat out on Al's postage-stamp balcony, wrapped in Terry cloth robes and wool blankets, drinking coffee and smoking early morning cigarettes. They sat in silence for a while, enjoying the buzz as it buffered them from the cold morning air. Al pulled Maggie's feet into her lap and rested a hand on her calf. She gave it a slight squeeze and held it, indenting impressions of her fingers into Maggie's soft flesh.

"Alaskan Salmon Fishing," Al said cryptically.

"Excuse me?" Maggie took a drag and coughed a little, her lungs out of practice.

"Exit strategy," Al clarified.

"Exit strategy?"

"Everybody needs one, Mags. Doesn't fishing sound nice? Honest work, something to show for it, a clear goal. Not too many people involved. Just you, the ocean, and the pursuit of fish. Like *Moby Dick*. What about you?"

"I hadn't thought about it."

"Hadn't thought about it? Hadn't *thought* about it?"

"I really hadn't. No imagination, I guess. Fishing sounds good, though. Little smelly, maybe. And I can't say I'm a fan of boats, now that I think about it."

"Only room for one burned out doc on the boat, anyhow."

"Yeah, I guess fishing is out for me."

Al drained her coffee quickly and went inside to pour herself another cup, leaving Maggie alone on the balcony for a moment. They were five floors up, and she was feeling that spaghetti-feeling in her legs that she often got at height, picturing a catastrophic strut failure of the balcony supports as the platform vibrated beneath her with the force of Al closing the sliding door behind her. Maggie pictured an eagle flying by at just the right moment and grabbing her like a kitten by the scruff of her neck to carry her away. Al returned before that could happen, and they sat in more silence.

"Maybe *this* was my exit strategy," Maggie said, breaking it. "Maybe I just won't go back."

Maggie lifted her eyes up from the coffee cup and made eye contact with Al, squeezing the sides of her eyes just enough to suggest a lightness to this statement, as if it could be a joke or not a joke, depending on the attitude of the receiver. Al reached over to grab Maggie's hand, a manner of intimate contact that — in spite of what had transpired the night before — seemed like it had broken through the glass wall that had always stood between them. She looked straight into Maggie's eyes, and opened her mouth as if to say something, and then closed it again, shaking her head.

"I know, I know, you don't shit where you eat." Maggie forced the corners of her lips into a wry smile that she hoped made her look casual and aloof. Alice continued shaking her head.

"You know, it's exactly the opposite? I'm the shit. It's me. I'm the shit."

Al's face was dead serious, but Maggie kept her smile up and squeezed Al's hand.

"What if I told you I eat pieces of shit like you for breakfast?"

"Are you really quoting *Happy Gilmore* right now?" Al took her hand back, laughing. This felt like a success to Maggie, making Al laugh, keeping the smile on her face, being clever instead of sad.

"You know," Maggie said, "I think being a novelist sounds good. Smutty romance novels about big muscly doctors and their damsels in distress."

"Nooow we're talking!"

Al patted Maggie on the knee, pushed her chair back, and stood up.

"Excuse me, I gotta shower. Too sweaty from last night, you know?" Al excused herself back into the apartment, turning back for a second and flashing her blue eyes at Maggie with a twinkle. Was that a slight bit of a *join-me* wink as she closed the sliding door behind her? Maggie didn't want to assume.

She considered trailing Al inside, but suddenly found her body to be leaden and unmoving, so instead she sat on the balcony, looking out at the city street and its movement and its trash and its liveliness and its young people with thin ankles walking their little dogs and carrying coffee cups like they are all in a movie about life in the city. She looked down at her own ankles, pale and swollen, and noticed how her belly hung out over her lap just so, and how the skin on her knees was forming little surface level spider veins that were highly visible in this morning light. She thought of Al, her body so lean and firm, as if it might just do a pull-up at any moment. She shook her head and got up, saying just audibly *you idiot* to herself as she walked inside. Inside, Maggie could hear Al humming a little tune in the shower, taking her time. The bathroom door had been left open, and the escaping steam had put the room into a softer focus.

Maggie quickly got her own clothes back on, pulling them on under her robe so as not to expose any unneeded flesh to her own critical eyes. When that was done, she slung her bag over her shoulder. It was heavier than she'd expected, and she remembered she'd brought Al a gift.

Maggie stepped softly into Al's bedroom, past the bed with its tangle of sheets in drunken disarray, over to the bedside table. She reached into her bag to remove the gift, giving it a little shake before she set it down on the table. She regarded it for a moment, then crept back to the door, slipping out and shutting it gently behind her. As her feet skipped down the exit stairwell, she sent a text: *Had to leave, but we should do this again sometime.*

Maggie had thought of it as simply polite at the time rather than a real proposition, and it hadn't gotten an immediate response. A few weeks later, Al had sent a photo of a woman holding two coconuts in front of her chest with the caption: *yes, we should do that again, sometime.* Maggie had replied with a *gif* of Shooter McGavin saying *I eat pieces of shit like you for breakfast,* and a winking emoji. A month after that, when elective surgeries had all been canceled during lockdown and surgeons were suddenly finding themselves on furlough, Al had driven the 700 miles to Missouri for a weekend, and a pattern was established. Sometimes there would be a real conference in Portland and Maggie would convince Christopher she should attend, sometimes it would be a furtive hotel room in Kansas City while Christopher worked a night shift, and it was always at least a few months apart. They always ended the same way, with a cigarette, an unspoken exit, a period of radio silence, eventually a little joke, and back to the beginning.

Afterward, Maggie would always return to Christopher, the Chief of Medicine, and she would get back to work. That was, until the incident.

CHAPTER 11

PGY9

The day of the incident, Maggie was standing in the stairwell. She was alone. Her head was leaned back against the wall, and her ponytail band was pushing into the base of her skull uncomfortably, but she made no adjustment. Her pager buzzed in her pocket, the single buzz to remind her of the previous buzzes she hadn't yet attended to.

She ignored it. Instead, she felt into her pocket for the presence of a certain box. She knew she didn't have time for it right now, being eight floors and four new admits and seven morning notes away, but just knowing it was there was enough to squeeze out a little juice into the right part of her brain. *Maybe I could* — the pager buzzed again — *or maybe not.* Maggie tilted her head forward, lifting it just off the wall, and the spot where her ponytail band had been digging in throbbed with its release. Maggie closed her eyes and thrust her head back into the wall again with just enough *zzuzh* to cause a momentary shock wave at the same spot. Buzz, went the pager. Buzz.

She could catalog the insults of the day, but for what reason? Nothing was that remarkable. People were dying, but people die every day, all over the world. It is literally inevitable, one of the two certain things in the world. So what? So what. People were mad, often at her, but so what? People get mad at grocery store cashiers, and babies, and little old ladies crossing the street too slow. Who was she to be spared? Computers were too slow. Supply closets weren't stocked. Potassiums were too low or too high. Urine output was meager. Nurses were paging her either too soon or too late for her liking. So what? The system was a dripping faucet, and Maggie a water balloon stretched beneath it, meant to just keep expanding.

The fact of the people dying wasn't new, of course, but the pace of it was growing old. They (whoever makes these decisions) were calling this *The Surge*, as if this term weren't delicately close to referencing the name of a horror movie about violently purging excess lives from the overburdened Earth. The people dying were patients, older ones, younger ones, often ones with *pre-existing conditions* that made her feel somehow safe, as if their risk factors were an inoculation against her own tragic demise; sometimes ones without pre-existing conditions would die too, and she would be reminded of the unfortunate chaos of everything around her. The people dying were colleagues sometimes, deaths that would make her say, *there but for the grace of god* before she remembered that she no longer believed in that kind of thing. The people dying were sometimes cantankerous public figures who had it coming, deaths that made her feel that uncomfortable gladness she knew she wasn't supposed to feel, but that she did feel, anyway. The same gladness she would feel when the families of end stage Alzheimer's patients finally agreed to hospice after cycles of increasingly futile hospital admissions for rehydration. Deaths that decreased the overall burden of suffering in the world.

When the incident started, it sounded like fireworks, and Maggie had rolled her eyes and thought, *jeez they're starting this patriotic shit early this year.* It then occurred to her that she was indoors, and the noises were likewise indoors, and that this would be an odd choice for an early Fourth of July celebration, wouldn't it? A doctor is a master of deductive reasoning, after all. She eventually arrived at the right logical destination, one she had been encouraged to arrive at by a number of required in-service trainings on the subject. If you hear hoofbeats, think horses. If you hear fireworks, and you are indoors, and it is not a patriotic holiday and you are not at Disneyland, think *Run, Hide, Fight.*

Maggie did none of those things. Though she felt her pulse rise, her body remained still, her eyes remained closed, and she took a deep breath in and held it. As she stood inert, she heard the stairwell door one floor below her burst open with yelling and crying voices and a thundering of feet shuttling themselves down, away from her and towards the exit, and then a similar burst from the floor below that, and the floor below that. She probably heard *Code Silver* come across a loudspeaker at some point, (as if this were a situation in which secret codes might be helpful), but her ears were ringing from the other sounds and she didn't register it. She knew what was happening, though, of course. She couldn't *not* know. A person knows in this part of the country, in this political climate, gun laws being what they are, the long arc of human nature bending as it has these days away from justice and toward destruction.

Still, in this knowing, she didn't move. Her head remained against the concrete wall, the cool concrete soothing the headache that was building from the excess pressure on her scalp from the ponytail band. Her breath must have gone in and out, since she remained conscious, but she had no recollection of having taken that air.

A mental health professional would later suggest to her that she must have been in shock; *we see it with soldiers in battle all the time, Dr. Owens.* She wasn't in shock, though. If anything, she was at peace. She listened as the fireworks got closer and closer, until eventually they came bursting through the door, one floor below her, following the footsteps of the people she had heard just a minute before. There was a pause, maybe just a couple of seconds, and Maggie felt something surprising. It wasn't fear, though she was holding her breath, though her heart was pounding, these were things her body was doing, but these were not her feelings. Her feeling — her feeling was relief. In the vacuum of that silence, her neglected pager buzzed again that single buzz, and to her it sounded like it echoed off the concrete corners of the stairwell like thunder. *Here it comes,* she thought. *Here it comes for sure.*

But it didn't. Instead of up, the footsteps went down, down, down, down, and then pushed their way into another door, and grew more and more distant, and then some different pops went off, and there was silence again. An acrid sulfur and singed-hair smoke rose upward in the stairwell into her nose, and Maggie felt her dread creeping back in. Her pager buzzed again. And it buzzed again. And she sat down. She reached into her pocket, and pulled out the box of cigarettes, and smiled. She lit up, right there in the stairwell, because what is a smoke in a hospital stairwell if the normal order of humanity has been torn asunder? She took a long and satisfied drag, and she waited.

Chapter 12

PGY10

After work, Maggie had agreed to meet Jess for a drink, to catch up and speak more frankly outside the prying eyes of the hospital building and its many cameras and busybodies. Jess had suggested a place a few blocks from the hospital, not far from her condo, for convenience. As Maggie walked out of the hospital and into the evening sun, she looked down at her watch, asking it the most important question: *Is there time for a cigarette?*

Just enough, the watch answered back, and Maggie walked with an eye into every alley on her way to the bar, finding at last a tucked-away spot between a pet food store and a high-rise retirement community that was unused and could provide shelter. As she stood, puffing with speed and efficiency, she looked out at the two competing streams of people passing her by. Fast walkers headed to the hospital, eyes down at the ground. Slower walkers headed towards the bars and restaurants, leaden with the gravity of the day, tides that went in and out as Maggie stood on the beach.

Look like hamsters spinnin' a wheel if you ask me, said Frank, puffing on his own cigarette beside Maggie.

Frank was right. This stretch of waterfront always had the feel, to Maggie, of a planned retirement community in which all the residents just happen to still be working. Instead of bingo and cha-cha lessons and badminton, the residents here all recreate with internal medicine and cardiology and surgery, and their communal cafeteria is a collection of drinking establishments that stretch like connective tissue between the condo buildings that hold everyone's bedrooms. If you were a certain kind of person in a certain stage of life, you could find yourself circling around and around this ten-block radius, filling up your bank account at the apex, emptying it at the zenith; filling up your belly on one side, emptying it on the other. The system providing for you, and you for it, in perfect symbiosis. Maggie put her cigarette out on the bottom of her shoe and stepped out of the alley to head the few blocks to the bar.

The Bitter End was a sprawling multi-story brewery positioned a few blocks southeast of Ella, on the waterfront proper with an outdoor second floor patio that looked out over the river and onto worn industrial buildings and ramshackle apartment complexes on the other side of the city, the side of the city not fueled by healthcare money or sneaker wealth and thus abandoned to the forces of decay.

Maggie grabbed a beer at the bar and headed out to the patio, taking a seat facing south. She was reminded of a visit she took once to the border town of El Paso, for a medical conference, where she had looked from the beige tones of that American city across the Rio Grande and into the splash of color that is Juarez, Mexico. Somehow, the rich side had the beige, and slums were like a rainbow. Water always seemed to create these yins and yangs where it ran, as if it were somehow the nature of water to split the fabric of society into competing parts.

Here Maggie sat on the side of yin, drinking a 9% IPA a little too fast and waiting for Jess to arrive, looking out on the view of the yang and thinking how odd it was that she should end up on this side of it. A cloud of vape smoke circled up from the mouth of a young man in a far corner by the balcony railing, not so far from her that she couldn't smell its combination of vanilla and mint, and sparking that certain type of yearning only known to unrequited lovers and unfilled nicotine receptors. She checked her watch and noted that Jess was seven minutes late, and asked the watch again. *Is there?* Her smoker's brain looked longingly out at her from across the river, beckoning her to join the other side. *Is there time?* Eight minutes late.

You just gonna sit here like an idiot? Frank was drumming his overlong nails on the table beside her. *Frank T. Blood don't wait, you know. Especially not for no broad.*

Maggie didn't answer. Instead, she took a deep, expansive breath in hopes of capturing some tiny fraction of her neighbor's vape cloud into her lungs, and pretended this might get just enough nicotine to sustain her. Around her, here in the aura of the hospital, were a sea of scrub-pant-wearing post-shift drinkers, chatting and drinking and flirting and not-flirting.

Maggie caught snippets of a conversation that was happening just at the edge of earshot. Maggie guessed the talkers were scrub techs, based on the words she could hear and the profiling she could gather by age and fashion and body habitus.

Kaufmann always complains [unintelligible] 16 French. He's such a fucking hack. [Raucous laughter] Did you get a load of that fat medical student? [Unintelligible] to make him cry.

Maggie was considering the ethics of trying to sit either closer or further away, when she spotted Jess stepping out onto the patio, looking like a vision in a cream pants-suit, punctuated by those heels with the pointy toe box Maggie couldn't imagine wearing but that some women seem to tolerate. Maggie supposed Jess must have been late on account of having to get this look together. *I take it back,* said Frank, letting out a low whistle, *this one might be worth waiting for.* Jess had a chilled white wine in hand, condensation glistening off the side of the glass in the indirect blush of eastern-facing evening light.

Maggie waved her hand up in the air to catch Jess' attention.

I just treat them like they are gnats, Maggie heard behind her other shoulder from the post-op table, followed by *ugh, enough work talk, we always talk about work. Did you watch The Bachelor last night?*

Jess waved back and weaved through the tables to take the seat across from Maggie. They didn't bother with greetings, as two people whose first meeting involved stripping naked in a locker room often didn't.

"Mags, I had a *day,* I tell ya." Jess was speaking in an insistent whisper, looking over both shoulders before continuing on. "Nothing but VIPs with mild dermatitis and wealthy white ladies who think every seborrheic keratosis is skin cancer, Jesus Christ. Not that I mind the RVUs, of course, but still. Sometimes I dream about pemphigoid or Stevens-Johnson syndrome, you know?" Jess took a drink from Maggie's glass before Maggie could stop her, and made a bitter face. "What the hell are you drinking, girl?"

Maggie slid her glass back toward her own chest and placed a protective hand on it. "I think it's called a StoneThrower. I like bitter beer, reminds me I'm alive." Maggie took another sip and recoiled a bit, realizing just now that she did not actually like bitter beer; the line about feeling alive was something Christopher had said and she'd adopted. She eyed Jess' white wine with envy and changed the subject.

"I had a metastatic cancer and an arson lung today, if you want to know what body medicine is like these days. You should join us if you're bored."

Jess made a *yuck* face and took a sip of her wine, as if to wash down the taste of what Maggie had said. "Double gross. Did you have to ask them about their poop? I feel like medicine doctors are always asking people about their poop."

Maggie shrugged. "Poop is the fifth vital sign, you know."

Jess laughed generously at what was not really even a joke. "I would have thought you and Al had enough of that kind of thing in first year, but I guess not." Jess's smile faded as Maggie's face fell, and Jess realized she had just summoned a ghost between them. "I'm sorry, I guess that's still kinda fresh for you."

Maggie took a big drink, her sinuses burning with hops and alcohol and carbon gas.

What're you waitin' for? Frank whispered in her ear. *Let her have it.* Frank was having the cigarette that Maggie couldn't have, sitting in an empty seat at the scrub-tech table. *You know you want to.*

"Jess," Maggie said, "I've gotta show you something." Maggie took a big gulp of beer, wincing as she held in a belch until it worked its way back down. Jess, as a counterpoint, was taking small, almost imperceptible sips from her wine, but on the periodicity of an IV drip. Sip. Pause. Pause. Sip. Pause. Pause. Where a third pause might sit, Jess spoke.

"Not a conspiracy theory, Maggie." Sip. Pause. Pause. "Please, not another conspiracy theory."

"Just *look.*" Maggie pulled up a message that she'd received on her way over, one that had caused her to gasp and cover her mouth in the universal sign of shock and awe when she'd opened it, one that caused her pulse to quicken now when she saw it again. She held her phone out to Jess, saying with an edge: "*I told you,* she's not dead. I *knew* she couldn't be dead."

From: jaxinyourbox@anonymous.net
Subject: Alice Power

As promised, here's your info.
Alice Power signed a lease for an apartment at this address six months ago:
10440 Highway 101
Brookings, OR
She received at least one paycheck from West Coast Fisheries, Incorporated, three months ago.
She voted in the last election.
Her car insurance is through Geico, and it's active.
She doesn't have a brother.
I couldn't find a death certificate under that name.
Thanks for the medicine, feeling so much better.

Jax

Jess's eyebrows tried so, so hard to raise while she took in this information. "What the fuck is this? Did you hire a private investigator in the time since our lunch break?" Jess's wine-sipping pattern quickened from 2:1 to 1:1. Sip, pause, sip, pause. Sometimes an extrasystolic sip-sip-pause snuck in between. Maggie was still gulping, feeling the forgotten effects of high-ABV west-coast IPA from which she had too long been separated.

"Better than a private investigator," Maggie said. "A youth. They might be a hacker. One of my patients on the ward today is one of those Burning Man chasers. You know about these guys? Apparently they got some kind of AI whoosiwhatsit, deep learning or oracle or something, I don't know how it works. I asked them to help me and it took 'em no time at all."

"*Maggie.* You asked a patient? To look for Alice? On the *internet?*" Jess had heard the words, but couldn't reconcile the usual decorum of medicine with this information, so she just kept repeating it. "A *patient.* You asked a patient. Like, one that is admitted to the hospital? For a personal favor? What was the part about 'thanks for the medicine,' anyway?"

Jess's face was one of both betrayal and curiosity. The way a prisoner looks at a plate of food that has been shoved through a door slot.

That's called investigatin' is what that's called. What's this broad's problem, anyhow? You got the lead, didn't you? Frank was blowing his smoke into rings that were widening and widening as they rose into the atmosphere, a skill that Maggie had always wanted to have but could never seem to achieve.

It just-then dawned on Maggie that her earlier stroke of genius may seem *indelicate* to an outside observer. She thought of the spreadsheet of lost licenses and medical board rebukes she had dug through the night before, searching for any cases that seemed similar. What was a tiny request for help finding a missing person when there were doctors defecating on the surgical trays and self-anesthetizing with halothane during off hours? What is a possibly borderline-unprofessional exchange of information done innocently in a helpful spirit, when there are other people retaining their licenses after having exchanged sexual favors for fentanyl patch prescriptions? Or is this the line of thinking upon which all of those other doctors first embarked upon their misadventures? A brief upward turn found its way to Maggie's lips as she imagined leaving a steaming turd on DoCTR Debbie's desk after-hours.

"I mean," Maggie said, hoping she wouldn't look back at this as the moment where everything changed, "it's not like I traded it for sex. They *wanted* to help." *And I would have ordered that oxycodone anyway,* she thought. Maggie believed that to be true. She was pretty sure she believed it to be true. She wanted to believe it was true, anyhow.

There was a silence as the two focused on their respective drinks. Sip, sip, sip, pause. Sip, sip, sip, pause. (Gulp). Maggie became increasingly disgusted with her beer, and eventually pushed it away, gazing out into the distance. The silence allowed nearby conversations to find their way back into Maggie's consciousness.

Oh my god, Kira is the Worst, the scrub techs were saying behind them. Maggie recognized it as *Bachelor* TV talk. *The absolute worst. What could Clayton possibly see in her? But what do you expect from a fucking doctor, right?* Jess slid the phone back across the table to Maggie.

"You really think it's Alice?" Her face had softened a bit, but was still circumspect. "And what if she doesn't *want* to be found, Maggie?"

Everybody wants to be found, Frank said. *Especially people who are hiding.*

"That's ridiculous, Jess. Of *course* she wants to be found. Why would she be leaving clues if she didn't?" Maggie reviewed the clues again. The voicemail, the phone call, the three dots, the new address, the obviously staged SocialEyes message. "I'll bet it's just a prank that went too far."

"I guess that sounds like Al," Jess conceded.

"Doesn't it, though?" Maggie and Jess had found at least a point of agreement, that this was something that was *like* Al, even if they didn't necessarily agree on the point that it was *actually* Al. Jess took another drink as Maggie looked on. Sip. Pause. Pause. The conversation at the scrub tech table boiled back over into earshot.

God, can you imagine anything worse than a fat doctor, the scrub tech was saying, apparently unable to let go of this bone. *Like, get a little self respect or something. Can't you get one of your buddies to prescribe you Ozempic already?* Maggie's ears started to turn red.

Haha, another one replied, *can you imagine taking health advice from someone like that? Jesus Christ.*

The whole table erupted in raucous laughter, and Maggie turned to them and stood up. "HEY," she said. The table was closer than Maggie had imagined, and she was surprised at the force with which this interjection came out of her. "HEY, HEY, HEY." The three people sitting there turned to look at Maggie, blowing out their vape smoke in her direction in near-unison.

"Yeah?" said a twenty-something young man with a buzz cut, sitting back in his chair with his legs crossed. "Can I help you?"

"You got a problem with FAT doctors, asshole?" Maggie said, one hand clenched into a fist by her side, the other patting at her own soft belly. "Hope your skinny ass doesn't end up on MY service, right?"

That erupted from Maggie's mouth as if she were a medium at a seance, transmitting a message from the beyond to a shocked audience. Surely it hadn't come from Maggie herself, who hated confrontation of any kind. Her face was already apologizing as she looked over at Jess, who was sipping, and sipping, and sipping, eyebrows still trying to be raised, forehead as smooth as a pearl. She wouldn't get involved. Maggie looked back at the table of scrub techs. She tried to even out the tone in her voice, to take out the shrill vibrations of her emotion, to be cool, and pleasant, and agreeable.

"Maybe," she said in this tone, glad to have her own self back, "maybe, you could *consider* thinking of these people as human beings, who are just doing their best, right?" Maggie took another deep breath, eyeing the half-smirk on the vape guy's face as he puffed vape smoke right at her. "Or maybe, if you can't do that, you can shut the *FUCK UP.*" In a sweet tone, though, with a smile.

Frank stood up and clapped, like a proud father at his child's dance recital. Around them, heads were turned in all directions at the noise. The scrub techs looked back at her, then at each other, then back at her.

"Hey, uhhhh, sorry," the vape guy, who seemed to be the ringleader, said to her.

Maggie's hands were shaking, and she turned around and sat back down before anyone could see it, turning her attention back to a shocked Jess, who was sipping, and sipping, and sipping.

She's not even that fat, Maggie heard the ringleader whisper to his neighbor.

"Um, are you *okay*, Maggie?" Jess was speaking quietly, to avoid being overheard by the scrub techs, who were now also speaking quietly, to avoid being overheard by Jess and Maggie.

"I. . .I don't think so. Nope, no, I don't really think I am." Maggie was reaching into her bag to pull out her smokes. She tapped one out and lit up. "In fact, I know I'm not." She took care to blow her smoke such that the wind would take it in the direction of her new enemies. "Do you sometimes just dream about taking a shit in broad daylight?"

Jess swallowed quickly to avoid spitting out her wine. "Um, no?"

"You know I don't even know why I became a doctor? I can't give even one good reason. I didn't have to. I just sort of. . .did. Like, by default. I showed up to med school thinking it was going to be this fun adventure, like a summer camp for altruistic nerds. And now I *literally* can't do anything else. Not a single other skill. Somehow my two options are to be a doctor, or to like, scrub toilets or bag groceries. I don't think I can even flip a burger at this point."

"What are you going to do? You can't quit, you know. They'll take back your signing bonus."

"Yeah," Maggie said. "I'll have to sleep on it, I guess."

Maggie's watch buzzed, an incoming email. She rolled her eyes when she saw the heading. Against her better judgment, Maggie scrolled down to read it.

From: deborahc@puh.edu
Subject: re: [ACTION NEEDED] Signature Overdue

Hi Maggie! Just a super quick reminder that we never got that pesky signature, so we've had to suspend your log-in! It's so super quick, just come on up and see us and we'll get your privileges reinstated!

Cheers!
Deborah Crockett, BA, MS, SHRM-CP, SSBB, PMP

Orientation Specialist
Department of Caregiver Training and Resources (DoCTR)

- Never doubt that a small group of dedicated people can change the world. Indeed it is the only thing that ever has - Mahatma Gandhi

This bitch, said Frank, *has some kinda nerve. My line of work, that kinda audacity and you'd be shaking hands with the sharp end of a blade if you catch my drift.*

Maggie took a cleansing breath and closed her eyes, visualizing her watch thrown high in the air over the city. At its apex, a falcon swooped down to pluck it out of the sky, then dove kamikaze into the sound to deposit it in the undertow, where it was carried out to sea. Maggie began to laugh a loud belly laugh, her soft belly shaking up and down like a jellyfish on a waterbed. "You know what, Jess? I know exactly what I'm going to do. I know *exactly* what I'm going to do." With that, Maggie downed the rest of her beer, swearing to never drink another IPA ever again, and pulled out her phone to consult a map. "Frank and I are going on the road."

Jess, again, almost spit out her wine. It was a bit she was doing, Maggie now realized. "Frank? What does Frank have to do with it?"

Maggie smiled a secret little smile to herself as Jess looked on. Then, Maggie began to sing: *"We all live in the House of Blood and Gas, we'll never get a pass, Frank T is on your ass!"*

Jess mouthed along with the remainder of the words silently, worry lines finding their way onto her usually pristine forehead as she did. *"He'll never really die, he'll never really die, he'll blow it up and take you down but He. Will. Ne. Ver. Diiiiie!"*

Jess laughed in that way you laugh when something isn't funny but rather odd. "Mags, I don't know what's going on with you, but I hope you find what you're looking for."

"Don't you worry, little lady," said either Maggie, or Frank, or both, "Frank T. Blood *always* finds what he's looking for."

Rise and shine, sweetie, Frank had awoken Maggie the next morning from a dream she had been having about him in a cheerleading outfit, cheering on a football team full of half-dissected cadavers. She sat bolt upright, and checked her watch: four AM. *Early bird gets the worm,* said Frank, *up and at 'em! Early worm gets the fish, too!*

She wasn't headed into the hospital this morning, as she'd decided the night before she had other plans for the day, and had responded to DoCTR Debbie's email with a curt apology that she wouldn't be able to get that form signed after all, owing to unforeseen circumstances. Instead, she threw on casual clothes, skipped the shower, and pulled her car out of the condo's garage for the first time since she'd parked it there a month ago.

Before she left, she turned to Frank and said, as directly as a midwestern woman could muster, "No offense, Frank, but this is just one of those trips a gal's just got to make alone."

Frank, not a man to stick around where he ain't wanted, turned heel and walked out through the wall, and Maggie was left again to her own thoughts.

The drive to Gold Beach could take one of two forms, depending on the heat with which you were traveling and your tolerance for winding coastal roads. Maggie, measuring high on the X-axis of the equation but asymptotic-to-zero on the y-axis, took the longer inland route on cruise control, listening to the latest episode of *Burn Report* on the way to pass the time. *Today we catalog the cost of Burning Man's reign of non-terror, trying to answer the question — is he a good guy, or a bad guy?* Listed in the good guy column was the measurable decrease in the city's landfill burden over the last year, as trash heaps meant for its subterranean grave were instead redirected skyward to a more heavenly fate. *City official Mark Lutz estimates Burning Man has saved the city at least 1.5 million dollars in waste processing costs over the last year.*

On her left, the sun was just peeking over the horizon, and on her right, an exit sign advertised that she might "Exit Now for *The Metal Detector Museum!*" and she considered the stop for the way back, given the trip's theme of hidden treasure. On the dash, the touch-screen flashed to let her know she'd just received a message back from

DoCTR Debbie, no doubt reminding her of the escalating consequences for each passing day of signature non-completion. Maggie got a little thrill thinking about Debbie marching up to the Green Team workroom, only to discover Maggie was missing altogether. Would her impromptu day off come back to bite her? In truth, she hoped it would. She imagined her name on the medical board website: *Licensee did willfully neglect the completion of life-saving onboarding modules, in violation of statute ORS 43.212 requiring physician subjugation at all times.*

Here, driving seventy miles-per-hour at the break of day away from the belly of the beast, she was not the system, and though the system could still find her here, it could not contain her.

On the other hand, her podcast host was saying, *fire crews have spent at least that much on overtime for a beleaguered fire-fighting force that have also had to contend with wildfires since the start of summer.* On Maggie's left, the sun found a way even from a billion miles away to reflect off the rear-view mirror and straight into her eyeballs, prompting her to tilt the mirror away. On the right, advertisements for gun shops and triple-X video stores were juxtaposed against signs for mega-churches and fetal heart-beats and the end times, all of which somehow co-existed happily in the zeitgeist down here.

But on the other, other hand, the podcast continued, *we could do worse than spending our money on fire-fighters.*

When she reached the southern part of the state, the route cut through a mountain pass to get to the coast, and she made it through that part with her fingers gripping the wheel, urging her arms not to give in to the impulse to steer the car off the side of the cliff, you know the one, the intrusive *what-if* that we all have in some measure when confronted with the opportunity to make friends with the abyss. As she came around the final curve, past a sign advertising a *Real Tiger Safari Park* that she filed away for later, the forest suddenly gave way to a broad and panoramic sky, and the wide expanse of ocean beneath it that had called so many retirees and social outcasts to these isolated and rocky hills.

From there, Maggie wound along the coast through the series of beach towns that were precariously built up in the tsunami zone, towns that perhaps fifty years from now would be buried under the sea like the lost cities of a modern climate-change Atlantis, but that for now sold fresh fish n' chips and used books and gave psychic readings and rented surf-boards to the crowds of rough-shod Oregon Coast surfers who would camp in conversion vans along the ocean-front. Eventually, Maggie's GPS led her down to a worn-out four-plex positioned next to an RV park just beyond the berm that separated the rocky beach from the coastal highway. In the parking lot, a single 90s-era Toyota Corolla sat with a rusted under-carriage, having somehow survived the great extinction event that had struck most used cars in the early 2000s. It would have stood out in the city, but made sense here in this place that still had no reliable cellular service, a fact that Maggie's phone was alerting her to now.

Here goes nothing, she thought, as she walked up to the door. The door, at one point, appeared to have been painted yellow, but as it faced the salt-spray of the water and the uninterrupted wind gusts that came from miles out into the open ocean, it was currently more of a gray-brown-mustard color that evoked baby poop more than sunny day. A plaque was positioned just underneath the doorbell that said *No Solicitors,* and Maggie paused for a second to consider if she was somehow captured in that exclusion, which she ultimately decided she was not.

She pushed the doorbell, and from inside the apartment she heard a harsh *brrrrrzzzh* go off, followed by a rustling on the other side of the door. There was a pause, and Maggie could see the shadow of an eye looking through the peephole on the other side, and she did her best to look non-threatening, realizing just at this moment that this was exactly the part of the state in which earlier this year a Jehovah's Witness was shot through the door by a scared *stand-your-ground*-er. The pause continued for longer than was comfortable, and Maggie felt compelled to say something.

"Hi, it's Maggie," she said. If it were Al on the other side of the door, it was information she surely already knew. If it were *not* Al on the other side of the door, the statement wouldn't make any sense at all. In that sense, she said it for no one, but it filled the silence.

"Maggie Owens," she added, also for no one's benefit. "I'm here to see Alice Power."

The door swung open, and Maggie stepped back a bit and grimaced in preparation for the worst. She was met with the sight of a slight, dark-haired woman holding a cup of coffee in one hand, gripping it in such a way as to suggest this would have been her weapon of choice had Maggie come with ill intention. Maggie held her hands up in front of her chest softly, to demonstrate she came in peace, and the woman relaxed.

"Hi, hello, hi," Maggie stuttered, moving slowly back in a way that was hopefully disarming and not suspicious. "Hello, good morning. I'm, I'm looking for Alice Power. Does she, does she live here?"

The woman's body relaxed a bit, though her eyes remained tense and narrow. She was wearing a shirt that said *2004 Buck'n Broncos Rodeo Rebellion* and booty shorts that were askew in a way that suggested she had just pulled them on in haste.

"No," the woman said. "She doesn't." She glanced behind her shoulder as she said this. Was it a tell? Was Alice hidden just on the other side of a bedroom door, having sent this woman out to *get whoever it is to scram*? Maggie tried to subtly peer over the woman's shoulder, but was too obvious and the woman tightened the angle of the door.

"Sorry, sorry. I'm just, I've come a long way, I'm trying to find her. Do you, do you know Al? Do you know where she is?" Maggie had parsed the woman's face when she had dropped Alice's name, and at the very least determined that most likely she knew Alice, based on the tiny smile that had escaped for a moment at the mention of her name.

"Oh, Al Power? I thought you said Alice for a second. Al Power ain't here either, though. She's not anywhere," the woman said. "Not anymore." Maggie understood the implication of this, but pretended she didn't.

"I'm a friend. I mean, I *was* a friend, or maybe I still am a friend, I'm not sure. But it's important that I find her." *Why is it so important* was a follow-up question that Maggie asked herself quietly in her own mind in follow-up, and she hoped that this woman would not pick it up, for Maggie had no answer for it other than, *because.* Maggie was shrinking her shoulders forward as she spoke, decreasing the target of her body such that the slings and arrows of follow-up questions may pass more easily around it should they come her way. "Or do you by chance know her brother? Brian?"

This prompted the woman to laugh out loud, a harsh and snorting belly laugh that erupted out of her small body and caused her un-supported morning breasts to bound up and down in a way that made Maggie cast her eyes away in embarrassment. The laughter went on past the point of comfort as Maggie looked on, and the woman's laughter cycles decayed into a long sigh and a wiping of invisible tears from her eyes. Maggie sat silently, with a Mona Lisa half-smile on her face, hoping the woman would find it unthreatening enough to explain.

"Sorry, sorry, sorry. I can't keep this up, I ain't no good at acting. Alice ain't got no brother," she said. "Brian Power is a made up person."

Maggie's eyes widened as she exclaimed, "I *knew* it. I *knew* Alice didn't have a brother!"

"Was her name really Alice? News to me. I only ever knew her as Al. Pretty sure that was on her driver's license."

Maggie cast her eyes down. "Oh, maybe she'd had it legally changed. Everyone did call her Al." This seemed important, a clue. *Jax had been looking for Alice, not Al.* Maggie raised her eyes back up to look at the woman. "So, wait, were you the person I sent messages to?"

"Guilty as charged," the woman said.

"Um, who are you, then?"

"Tiff. I, uh, well, I was kinda spending time with Al before she, well, you know."

Maggie's nose recoiled as she listened, and she swallowed hard. A smell of rot had wafted on the air and was making her eyes water.

"Oh?" Maggie coughed, urging the smell to pass before she was overcome by the urge to vomit. "Were you her roommate?"

"Well, I'd say I was more than a roommate," Tiff said with a wink. "But I was also a roommate."

"Oh," Maggie stuttered, "I see." It only just now occurred to

Maggie that she might feel jealousy at the thought of Al with another woman. Her reflex was immediately to size the woman up in comparison to herself. Tiff's face was pretty, with an angular nose, well-sculpted eyebrows, and perfectly-straight teeth, but she had a shadow under her cheeks and a hint of pink in the conjunctiva that suggested *something* to Maggie. A habit? A sadness? An eating disorder? Her hair and skin were worn down, and her hands looked rough, so Maggie could take those points in her own favor. Maggie tried to keep her face in the purposefully neutral look that she would use when examining a festering diabetic foot ulcer, a look that says *no judgment here, just curiosity.* "How long were you, um, *roommates?* Did you know her in Portland?" *Did she choose you over me, or did you come later?*

"Ha, me? No, no. I met Al on the boat, we worked together, brief as it was. Weird woman, you know? Not a lot of doctors working the deck on a fishing crew. I got a big-ass cut the first week out and she stitched me up, and I moved in the week after, you know how it is. She was funny you know? Everybody kinda liked her, the whole crew came to the funeral."

Maggie gasped at the word *funeral,* which made plain what Tiff had previously been talking around. Who could need a funeral but a dead person, and Al needed a funeral, and Al was dead. Al was dead. Al couldn't be dead, but Al was dead. Maggie suppressed a gag as Tiff kept talking.

"I mean, not really a funeral. More a memorial service. She was supposedly a doctor but she didn't seem to have any money, you know? So I got stuck tryna figure her shit out after the fact." Tiff had an inscrutable look on her face, something like a smile in the upper half that morphed into a forced frown in the lower half. "You know I kept hopin' someone would show up at some point, and here you are."

"Well, alright then, here I am. Can you tell me what happened?"

Tiff shrugged, eyes darting up and to the side, either in remembrance or in avoidance. "I guess it might have been an accident. I'll never know for sure. She didn't leave no note or anything. I think they called it an overdose, common enough around here so they just kind of assume. I just woke up and — well, *you know.*" Tiff kept saying *you know* in place of the exact piece of information that Maggie had wanted confirmed. "Medics took her wallet, ID, and everything. They never asked me for any more details and I never told 'em, neither. Her rich-ass family didn't give any kind of a shit about her, I guess maybe they'll figure it out eventually, maybe they won't."

Maggie was purposefully keeping her brain in investigative mode for this conversation, trying to channel herself as Frank T. Blood, hot on the final trail of a hard-boiled mystery, trying to keep her quickly-expanding emotions from bubbling out of her gut and escaping into the atmosphere. "And you, you must have been the one that sent a message to our medical school class? To the SocialEyes group?"

Tiff was nodding, nodding. Shrugging. Eyes to the ground.

"Yeah, that was me, alright. They came and took her away, and then I was just *here* in the apartment. I looked through her phone, didn't find no emergency contact, so I looked through her laptop and saw she'd been, like posting all that stuff there. So I sent that message, so people would know. You know? I just felt like I needed to tell someone. I thought maybe someone would get in touch, but no one did. Well, til' you I guess."

Maggie was putting pieces together in her mind. "Wait, so *you* are the one that has her phone? You are the one who called me? You are the one reading the texts?"

Tiff was nodding, apologetically, eyes cast down. "Yeah, guilty as charged. Like I said, I kept hopin' someone would show up. You know she owed me a lot of money? Said she was givin' all her money to lawyers. But the phone's on some kind of autopay. So's the rent. I figure why let it go to waste, you know what I mean, not like she's around to use it any longer. I guess eventually the money will run out and it'll get shut off and I'll get evicted."

"That makes sense, Tiff. I — I'm so sorry you had to deal with all this."

Tiff shrugged, in that way that Maggie had seen people shrug off death because they'd seen it so many times before. "Hey," Tiff said, "were you and Al, were you close? Like, you were friends?"

Were they close? Was it possible to ever be close to the sun? Sure, to you it feels close because the sun is so powerful and hot. But to the sun? You are just one of a million specks of dirt in orbit. Maggie didn't say all this, instead screwing up her face in that *maybe* way. That seemed good enough for Tiff, who got an aha look on her face.

"Hey, I got something that, I dunno, it belonged to her. Seemed kinda special, so I kept it, but maybe someone who knew her better should have it." Tiff closed the door and left Maggie standing there for several minutes, long enough that Maggie wondered if she was returning or if she had somehow snuck out a side door and was running away down the beach. Just as Maggie was about to walk around to peer in a side window, the door opened again, and Tiff presented Maggie with a snow globe. This snow globe was a particular snow globe, which at its base had the form of an ancient ruin, with the word POMPEII chiseled into its faux bricks. Within the globe itself, an erupting volcano. Maggie shook it, and the thick layer of gray glitter-ash that had been lying at the base of the globe erupted up in a circular and chaotic cloud. Underneath where the glitter-ash had been settled were tiny sculpted figurines with shocked and terrified faces, caught in a run for their lives they would never win, stuck forever in the stasis of this worst and last moment of their lives. Maggie and Tiff both stood in silence and watched as the circling ash settled down, covering the bodies slowly back up until all that was left was a peaceful and quiet landscape.

"Where did you find this?" Maggie said, holding the globe in her outstretched hand as if it were a baby bird that might take flight at any moment.

"It was on the nightstand. Kinda weird, right? She hardly had anything personal in her apartment, but she had this."

Maggie thanked Tiff for the globe, for her time, and stepped back to turn back to her car, when she realized a question that had been left unasked. *Frank T. Blood would never leave without closure,* she thought, and worked up the courage to ask it.

"Hey, I was hoping to maybe pay my respects. Do you know where, if you don't mind, what happened to, well, *you know.*"

"Her body?"

"Yeah, exactly." Maggie was glad to not have to say the word herself.

"*Well*, let me tell you honey, bein' dead is *not* cheap, you know? Even being cremated is, well, let's just say we don't have that kinda money in *this* household. And like I said, I didn't have *access* to her accounts. But the people who came, they said we could like, *donate* the body to science, and I thought for sure that's what a woman like that would want, right? She was some kinda doctor. So I signed her up for that. They said the school could get it, I thought that sounded pretty good."

Maggie took a moment to process this information.

"The school?"

"Yeah, you know them students gotta like, cut one up to learn on it? I signed her up for that. They're gonna cremate her for free when they're done. I guess one of these days I'll get her back on my doorstep in a little metal box, but it ain't happened yet."

"She's at the school? *Here?* Like, the school here? Up in the city?"

"Yeah! Seemed like, poetic right? Send her right back to where she came from?" Tiff looked right proud of herself, and was looking at Maggie as if she ought to be proud along with her. "I was jus' gonna like, scatter her into the ocean when she showed up, unless maybe you want to split her? You're the only one's showed up since she died."

"Wait, so the school *still* has her?" Maggie was stuck, skipping back in the vinyl of her mind to the same point. "Like, she's *still* there?"

Tiff nodded. "I guess it takes a while? I don't know, you'd probably know better than me, right?" Tiff shuddered, imagining some version of what was happening that was probably, actually, less grotesque than the reality. "It's been three months already," Tiff said, chuckling quietly. "Hope they got her in a freezer or somethin'. She gotta be *ripe* by now."

"Huh."

"Yeah."

The two women stood there for a full minute, Maggie's eyes cast at her own navel in reflection, Tiff's cast at Maggie's eyes in annoyed anticipation. When Maggie finally looked up she was startled to have the fullness of Tiff's gaze directed right at her eyeballs. Her eyes went back down.

"Oh! I'm sorry, I don't want to take any more of your time, I guess. You've been very gracious."

"Yeah, I have been, haven't I. Very gracious. Did you say you're a doctor too?" Tiff said, looking down at Maggie's bag by her side, the bag that contained the precious snow globe. "If you've got any way to help me out, you know, I'd appreciate it."

Maggie caught the hint, and reached in to grab her wallet, and went through the theater of showing that she was all out of cash. "Oh, it doesn't have to be cash," said Tiff, staring down Maggie as an eager cat might a passing bird. "I got Venmo, CashApp, ApplePay."

"Oh, sure, sure, sure. Happy to help you out Tiff, really I am. I know you've been through a lot."

"Great, my handle is @alaskanfisherlady if you wanna look me up." Tiff spelled it out for clarity.

"Alaska?" Maggie was scrolling through her phone apps to try and oblige Tiff, suddenly a little fearful at what would happen if she didn't.

"Yeah, that's where I work half the season. Up north on the big fishing rigs, salmon, crab, you know. Right now, well, it's been slow. That's why I could use the help."

Maggie was nodding along, and then stopped for a second.

"Did Al make it up to Alaska?"

"Doubt it. Not with me, anyway." Tiff's phone buzzed at her and she picked it up briefly. "Hey, thanks, thanks. That's generous of you. Appreciate it."

"Yeah," Maggie said, looking again over Tiff's shoulder and into the apartment, looking for a glimpse, of what she wasn't sure. A shadow? A ghost? She saw in Tiff's face that their time was through. "Gosh, thanks so much for your time, I appreciate it. Um, take care. Have a good day, thank you for your time." As if she were going door to door to sell solar panels or pest control services.

"Yeah, have a good day!" Tiff said cheerfully as she shut the door. Maggie heard the front door lock engage with a *snap* as she turned to walk back to the car. As she walked, her fingers fumbled to remove the keys from her pocket, her hand confused by the unsteady strides that her Danskos were taking on the undulating gravel of this beachfront driveway. Her hand, she realized, was shaking, and her fingers wouldn't grasp her Minnie Mouse key chain to pull it out, getting only handfuls of pocket lint.

The key chain had been a gift from her grandmother when Maggie was a teenager, given to her on her 16th birthday when she got her driver's license. Her grandmother had been under the impression that the teenaged Maggie had been holding a torch for Disney characters since her fifth birthday when she had requested a Minnie Mouse cake, and had continued giving Minnie-themed gifts until her death twelve years ago. The thought of her grandmother dug into her sadness, as she wished now she had been able to know the woman as a human being and not a source of unwanted gifts. *I'm sure she's in a good place,* Maggie thought, as the metal Minnie-head finally freed itself from her pocket and brought her fob key out with it.

It wasn't even necessary to have the key out, of course. Since the moment Maggie had walked away from it, the car had been sending out desperate pinging wavelengths in search of the key, *are you back, are you back, are you back now,* until Maggie and her pocket-key mercifully appeared within the range that auto-unlocked the doors. Still, Maggie felt compelled to push the button. In a world designed without friction, sometimes she just needed the feeling of it.

The drive back toward the city went by in silence; Maggie left the radio off. She'd placed the snow globe on the dash, wedged up against the windshield like a beacon. With each bump of the worn coastal roads the snow-globe ash would disturb in a flurry, uncovering the shocked human faces gazing up to the heavens, only to be slowly covered back over by the settled ash.

Along the hypnotic drive, Maggie thought of the real Mt. Vesuvius, famously erupting two thousand years ago, melting the faces of a thousand residents of Pompeii with a pyroclastic surge and a thirty-kilometer column of hot ash that preserved the cursed village perfectly for archaeological study. She thought of the real Mt. Vesuvius still standing, still erupting from time to time, violently, catastrophically. She thought of the 600,000 people still living in the shadow of the mountain, selling little snow globe souvenirs to tourists passing through, waiting for the next column of ash to either push them from their homes or kill them outright. *Will we ever learn from history? Even once?*

The car hit a bump, the ash flew up, the end was nigh. The road was smooth, the ash settled, it was over. Again, and again, and again. Eventually perhaps, there would be a last time.

Were there doctors in Pompeii? Men who had undertaken years of apprentice training, only to watch helplessly as the skin peeled off the entire city all at once? As their own skin peeled off with it? Sometimes, that's the job. To bear witness, even when it's unbearable.

Maggie wasn't thinking about any particular plan of action as she drove, just chain smoking and bouncing along with the ash, shaking off one reverie in favor of the other, over and over again until several hours later the car was winding up onto the hospital hill and pulling into a patient parking garage as if on autopilot. *Oh look,* she thought, *look at where I've ended up,* as if by surprise. She knew what she was doing here, of course, though she was pretending to herself she didn't. She put her last cigarette out in the soda cup serving as an ashtray in the center console, and didn't bother with her post-tobacco smell protocol. If anything, the stench might be helpful today.

Welcome back, doc, said Frank as Maggie shut the engine off. *You find what you were lookin' for out there?*

"You don't know the half of it, Frank," she said. "But I think you're going to want to see this."

Maggie scurried out of the garage and back into the sunlight, and Frank followed a few steps behind. It was the late afternoon, and there were quite a lot of people out on campus, spilled out over the green spaces, as a waning fall sun was luring any who could escape the hospital walls to do so. The outdoor benches were taken up by handfuls of late-lunching nurses and residents, taking a moment to replenish their vitamin D and their caffeine before returning to their respective grinds. Maggie pulled on a surgical mask, hoping to avoid recognition.

As she walked past the central courtyard fountain positioned between the parking garage and the main hospital, Maggie spotted Henry, the resident from the Green Team, lying in the grass. He was face up, arms outstretched to the side, with scrub sleeves rolled up above his deltoids to maximize the exposed surface area. His eyes were closed and his legs were straightened with his feet together, and it gave the overall impression of his being frozen in the middle of a serene high dive. Maggie's first instinct was to check for the rise of his chest wall. She stared long enough to get that proof of life, then scurried past to avoid catching his attention. A symphony of bullfrogs chirped in the near-distance, a reminder that this place was situated in the middle of a wilderness, in spite of all the trappings of urbanity.

Walking through the hospital was a different experience in street clothes, without the armor of her white coat to reflect the light. People seemed to look right through her, as if she were an extra in a movie, didn't move out of the way as she walked, didn't nod or smile at her. A hospital badge sat in the pocket of her bag, though, a secret key to the inner spaces of this place, and she ran her finger across the edge of it, wondering if it would bring her the access that she needed for where she was headed.

You gonna tell me where we're headed, said Frank, *or is it some kinda secret?*

"You'll see," said Maggie.

You know I won't, Frank responded, *on account of my eyeballs are missing.*

At 4 PM, the morgue level should be cleared of first year medical students, who would have wrapped up the day's dissection hours ago. There might be some surgical residents around, completing the exemplary prosection for the following day's structures, though if she knew surgical residents as she thought she did, they may not even notice the presence of an interloper in the lab, and if they did, they wouldn't have the energy to care. If needed, she could flash her badge at them. It had a hang tag on the bottom that said in large and bold lettering ATTENDING PHYSICIAN, which would surely strike fear in their hearts. What would she do once she was there? She wasn't sure. But she had come this far, right? She had come this far.

She passed by the Green Elevators, figuring that a secret mission is best not carried out in such a public-facing area, heading instead for the camera-less Faraday cage of the concrete stairwell around the corner. As she set down the stairs, she heard a group of deep voices echoing from above, voices descending toward her at a rate that she suspected meant they were tall and taking the stairs multiple at a time. The chatter suggested interventional radiology, as they volleyed about things like who had the best *door to groin puncture time* and other hospital speed records. *Get yourself a Model X,* the record-holder was saying, *it'll get you to the hospital faster and it's fucking real fun to drive up the hill and they let you park in front of the ER entrance.* Maggie made a decision to just slow up and let them pass her, rather than trying probably in vain to outrun them. *On your left,* one of them called out as they saw her ahead, as if they were cyclists on a track, and soon after they brushed past her on their way to wherever they were headed, the slight chemical perfume of chlorhexidine wafting by with them. A minute later, she heard a heavy door open and close, and the voices and footsteps disappeared. She picked her pace back up, and before she knew it was rounding the corner on the door for LEVEL M.

She slowed down for the last few steps, realizing she wasn't sure what she would do once she arrived at the door. Most other floors had doors with a window to view through the door (lest you take out the face of someone on the other side), but this one was solid steel, painted a flat and ominous black. There was a badge reader by the door, and an adjacent red-letter sign. *Restricted Access.* Everything about it suggested she should stop and reconsider the choice. *Turn back,* it was saying to her, *there be bodies in these hills. Be wary all you living people who should pass through here.* She wasn't even sure if her badge would open this door, and she was hesitant to try until she had decided if she was going to follow through with whatever it was she had planned. She could imagine very few reasons why an attending physician of her station would need to access the morgue floor, and so that would argue that it *shouldn't* work; on the other hand, the badge-access protocols rarely seemed to make that kind of sense in her experience, as she knew in medical school that her student badge often gave her access to supply closets that her attendings couldn't get into and a doctor's lounge that she was explicitly prohibited from entering, as if the point of the badge was entrapment rather than security. If it didn't let her through, she was facing both disappointment and the daunting trek back up the stairs. If it did let her through, she was faced with the reality of completing a macabre task she was surprised she was even considering. A badge swipe would be recorded, somewhere, would place a name to her anonymized mask-and-street-clothes incognito form, would allow some security guy somewhere (or, more likely these days, a security bot) who was tasked with monitoring Unauthorized Morgue Entries to make a note in her record. Perhaps DoCTR Debbie would get a text alert.

What're you waitin' for, doc? Get ON with it. No sense backing out NOW. Frank was smoking in the stairwell, and Maggie inhaled deeply as she stood contemplating. At the height of her inhalation, the door burst open, and she recoiled, both from the steel door that narrowly missed her nose and the smell that didn't. *Hey, watch it,* said Frank, as he stumbled backward onto the stairs. A couple most likely surgical residents had burst through the door and were equally startled by the encounter, making brief shocked eye contact with Maggie before casting their eyes down apologetically. One muttered a breathy apology, while the other held the door for her to go through, neither of them seeming to notice she was a clear interloper. This was as much a sign from the universe as any, she thought, and took the win. She ducked through the door and entered the hallway and the surround-sound-smell of formaldehyde wrapped around her as the door clunked shut behind her.

Wait a minute, said Frank, *wait ONE minute. Where the fuck are you taking me?*

"You'll see," said Maggie.

The hallway was empty, and the path to the dissection lab was now clear of any obstacles or observers. She started walking, thinking *I could turn back at any moment* followed by, *but I've come so far.* One foot, then another foot, taking her closer to what was certainly going to be an upsetting version of the closure she had been seeking. *Surely this was what Al would have wanted,* Maggie thought. *Or still wants, depending on what I find.*

She thought of Al, somehow posthumously aware of her location, laughing at the thought of her inguinal canal or her anal triangle or her bulbospongiosus being flayed open by scandalized twenty-some-things; at the thought of her face being peeled away by layers until just the bare bones remained, in a final metaphorical fuck you to the system.

You want me, Maggie pictured Al saying to the hospital and the medical system as a whole, *well, here I am you motherfuckers.*

She found herself standing at the door to the dissection lab, a door that would also have had a badge entry requirement if someone hadn't taped over the magnetized door latch with electrical tape. Maggie recognized this move from her own med school days, an unofficial part of the dissection protocol that had been passed down from years before her and now, apparently, to years after her as well. The gunners would do this to allow late-night entry into the lab, past the usual operating hours that were designated by the school, so they could furiously catalog the paths of brachial plexuses and branches of the celiac trunk, under the beneficial influence of prescribed and non-prescribed stimulants. Their professors knew the tape was there, of course, and never bothered it. *In my day, the students all slept in the anatomy lab so they could spend as long as possible with the source material,* they would probably say at some point during the course. This is the education of a doctor, as much as the names of the parts, how to give yourself up to the work.

Maggie peeked through the porthole window in the door to the lab and saw no living forms there to stop her from entering. She pushed the door open and she was inside, as if having been trans-ported in time, nothing having changed substantially from fourteen years ago.

The door closed behind her, and Frank remained on the other side. *You're on your own from here, doc. I ain't goin' in THERE again, no thank you,* he said, lighting a new cigarette and strolling back down the hallway and out of sight.

Maggie looked around the room. The tables were arranged in ten rows of three, each with a body covered by a now grimy off-white sheet. A clipboard hung on the end of each table, and below, a red bucket closed with a snapping lid. The saccharine chemical smell of formaldehyde hung everywhere around her. The smell was not as bad as she had recalled it being back then, perhaps the technology for preservation had come along, or perhaps her own smoking habit had diminished her perception of it, or perhaps both. She strolled along the rows, stopping to tilt the clipboards up to check the age of the cadaver, looking for one that was conspicuously younger than the rest. Five rows back, she found it.

Female, 38, the clipboard said. *Cause of death: Presumed Overdose.* The feet had been hastily covered such that the soles were peeking out on the end, cold, gray, plasticine. Maggie shivered from the refrigerated air in the room and stared at the feet for a moment, fighting an impulse to grasp them with her hands to warm them up as she might do if they were slung across her lap on a couch. She held back, knowing that to touch the body would be truly transgressive, but also feeling like, *I've come this far.*

She thought about looking around the room for cameras, but decided that assuming there *were* cameras, the act of scanning the room to *look* for them would surely be the most suspicious thing she could do. If there was one thing she had learned from heist movies, it was to *look like you belong.* So, she did just that. *What would Frank T. Blood do,* she thought, here in his ancestral home. She waited for Frank to say something to her, but he was long gone, so she filled in the blanks.

Frank T. Blood would get to work.

Maggie grabbed some gloves from the rack under the table, snapping them on confidently for show, like you see in a movie, like Al had done the day they'd met. She walked up to the head of the table, turned off all critical thought, and flung the top of the sheet back. The sheet's movement created a brief wind across her face that caused her to close her eyes briefly before sneaking them back open.

Somehow, in the bluster of all this confident movement, she hadn't thought about what was to come next. She had expected another layer of separation, based on her calculations, and was surprised to find the head un-shrouded, but also yet un-dissected. The eyelids were taped shut to cover what Maggie knew were cavernous holes where the eyes had been harvested for special preservation. Eyes that wouldn't sparkle at her as they told an off-color joke, because they were in a back freezer somewhere encased in some kind of preservative fluid. She tried to focus her own reluctant eyes on the form.

It was not Al. It couldn't be. The face was fallen, dour, sunken in a way that Al's face could never be, and the features seemed too small, too insignificant. On the other hand, there was a perfection in the eyebrows, there was a short-cropped stubble of black hair atop the head, there were trappings that could suggest an Al-shaped box. There were features that could be checked on a list of physical characteristics. Things a police sketch artist could recreate if needed. But it also wasn't Al. But perhaps it was? Al had no identifying tattoos, and neither did this person, but lots of people didn't, and so this was neither evidence for nor against. She thought of the piercing that Al had sported in one of her last SocialEyes photos, the one that traveled through her nasal septum. Maggie thought if she could look for a hole there, maybe she could know for sure. She reached out to turn the face toward her, cradling one cheek of Al-but-not-Al in her hand.

She had just started to lift up the tip of the nose for inspection when the door to the lab burst open. The surgical residents, having gone to grab afternoon coffee, had returned to complete their work. The noise caused a jump-scare in Maggie, who — because she was *not* in fact a seasoned private eye, but an easily frightened middle-aged woman — yelped, pulled her hand away, and tipped out of her precarious shoes all at once. This had two immediate consequences.

First, Maggie lost her footing and fell sideways, trying and failing to hold the table to steady herself, grabbing instead just the edge of the table along with a handful of sheet that ripped off as she tumbled over. Her head perfectly caught the corner of the adjacent table on the way down, finding that sweet spot on the skull base where boxers aren't allowed to punch on account of how easy a knockout it is, and she was rendered unconscious, slumping to the ground in a disorganized and undignified heap.

Second, the pull of Maggie's surprised hand against the cheek of Al-not-Al had knocked the lean body askew on the table, and her subsequent unraveling of the sheet-cover and tilting of the table's edge had rolled the body right over the edge, tumbling face-down onto the ground and to a final resting position atop the legs of a now-unconscious Maggie.

What the surgical residents were, let's be honest, delighted to find when they ran to the scene, was a crumpled Maggie, bleeding theatrically from her lacerated scalp, a handful of formaldehyde-soaked sheet in her left hand, breathing heavily and moaning in her concussed and unconscious state. They found Al-but-not-Al, face down to reveal the patchwork-quilt appearance of a dissection-in-progress, strips of cut paraspinous muscle falling out to the side, delicately defined nerve pathways now torn and hanging precariously, left elbow pointed awkwardly akimbo as the tendons that would normally hold it in line had been bagged in favor of deeper exploration.

Maggie started to come to after a moment, as she heard one of the residents saying *what the fuck* and another saying *hold the C-spine* and another saying *should I grab a stapler?* There was laughing. *Jeez, her lab partners are gonna be pissed.* She felt firm pressure squeezing her ears between two strong forearms as someone grasped her shoulders from above to prevent her from turning her head. She moaned and seemed to try to object, but found her mouth couldn't quite move.

"Baaah," she said as she opened her eyes to find a blurry face shining a pen light in her eyes and rubbing her sternum painfully. "Ow, that hurts," she finally managed to say.

Can you tell me your name, the resident was saying. *Can you tell me what day it is? Can you squeeze my finger?*

"Al, that's not funny," she said, squeezing the finger and pulling a bit as well. She was being pulled away from the body and laid back, and someone was pushing on the back of her neck. *Does this hurt? Does this? Does this?* Maggie tried to shake her head *no,* but found she couldn't. She had a tremendous headache and drifted back into sleep to escape it.

A halogen light intruded upon Maggie's sleepy eyelids as two fingers worked at prying them open.

"Oww, stop, I'm trying to sleep," she said to the light, to the fingers.

The light and the fingers did not listen. "Maggie," the light responded, "you're in the emergency room. Can you wake up?" The light had a second hand that was using its knuckles to rub painful circles upon her sternum. "Wake up, Maggie."

"God. Yeah. Whoa. What?" Maggie opened her eyes voluntarily now and found a masked face staring back down at her. The face was soon replaced again by the offensive light, which shone at point-blank range into her right eye, then left, then right, then left, swinging back and forth to interrogate the painful contractions of her pupils. Yes, interrogation was the right word, Maggie thought. Had she been arrested?

"You're in the emergency room," the voice said. "You've sustained a head injury. Can I ask you some questions?" Given this context, Maggie answered on instinct.

"Maggie Owens, Friday August 19th, University Hospital, one hundred, ninety-three, eighty-six, seventy-nine —"

The voice laughed, turned the light off, and put a hand on Maggie's arm. "Okay, okay, okay. Do you have any pain anywhere?" The voice was now resolving into a face, a young face, with blond curls and wire-rimmed glasses and a green binder peeking out of a white-coat pocket Maggie guessed meant the face belonged to a resident. The fingers had stopped prying at her eyes and were now poking the back of her neck, which she noted was currently enclosed by a rigid collar. Maggie reached her own fingers behind her head, to an area that she was noticing did have pain. A cold ridge of metal staples lined a track along the back of her head, and she pushed on them and winced.

"My head, it hurts. My head hurts," Maggie said, giving an accusatory glance at the resident. "There are staples in it."

"You hit your head, Maggie," the resident said. "You were bleeding." The resident offered no other apology. He was looking down at a checklist that he carried on a laminated card, and was trying to get answers. What is your name. Where are you. What is today's date. Even though these have been asked and answered, they need to be answered to the checklist as well. Maggie reiterated that her head hurt.

"Can you rate your pain on a scale of one to ten?"

No, Maggie wants to say. *Pain is not solid in that way. Pain is gaseous and expansive and slippery. Pain takes up the entire vessel, every time. Pain is both infinite and non-existent. Pain is a number, but it is not a real number, it is imaginary. My pain is the square root of negative one.* The masked, bespectacled face looked at her, looked at the checklist, looked at her.

"Seven," she answered, and the face was satisfied. "Um, my head hurts," Maggie said. "There are staples in it." The face patted her on the arm and turned his head over to someone else who was standing at a corner computer.

"C-spine is clear, GCS is fifteen, but she's perseverating," he said to the other person, who entered the information into Maggie's record. He peeled the collar off of her neck and said, "Let's get her five of oxycodone, and set her up for fifteen minute status checks." The face turned back to Maggie, putting a hand presumptuously on her arm and stroking lightly with a thumb. He talked to her in a voice that you used with a lost child. "Boy, you took quite a tumble! I think you'll be okay, though. We're going to call your emergency contact to come and pick you up, okay?" Maggie nodded in agreement, because what else could she do in this moment, a moment where her head hurt, and there were staples in it, and she was trying to piece together the other pertinent facts of the situation.

"Is Frank here?" she said, as a lingering smell stuck to her nose and jogged her memory. "No, wait, no. Frank can't be here. Or can he?" The resident and the other one (who knows, a nurse or another resident or an admissions officer) just looked at her with raised eyebrows. "Frank? Is that who I mean? Yeah, Frank! Is Frank here? Frank, are you here?"

There was no response from Frank. Insofar as Frank could have been there before, he seemed to be gone now, perhaps evicted permanently by the power of the blow. The unidentified person looked up from the computer. "It looks like your emergency contact is someone named Christopher? Is that right? Is that who you're looking for?"

"Christopher?"

Her head hurt. She reached up and confirmed again that there were staples in it. Why are there staples in her head? She retraced her steps that day. The drive to the hospital, the walk down the stairs, the swinging stairway door, the lab, *oh that's right, the lab,* and then the whole lot of it came flooding back to her at once.

Al. Al was dead. Or she wasn't. Al was alive, living on the south coast. Or she wasn't. She was in the dissection lab, or was it someone else. Al was a Burning Woman, or no Burning Woman existed, or Al was dead, or she wasn't. Al was both alive and dead at once, until Maggie could find the box that contained her and open it. Al was timeless, like the shocked and frozen faces of those snow-globe inhabitants, destined to die the same death over and over and over and over any time someone came to shake the globe.

Maggie heard her phone buzzing and buzzing and buzzing in her bag next to the bed, and she swung her legs over the side of the bed so she could reach it. *Christopher Lab Partner,* it said, perfectly on cue. She swiped right to answer.

"Hey," she said. "I guess the hospital probably called you."

"Maggie," Christopher said. "What the heck is going on? They told me some kind of crazy story about —"

"Yeah, yeah, I know. It's all true," Maggie said. "Also, my head hurts. They put *staples* in it."

"I booked a flight out, but I can't get there until tomorrow." Christopher was speaking to her in his professional voice, a voice of compassion and care and no judgment that was hard as hell to say no to. "I'm here for you, Maggie."

Maggie knew four things in that moment.

First, that her head hurt.

Second, that they had put staples in it.

Third, that Al was dead, or at the very least Maggie needed to accept she was.

Four, that Maggie was leaving this place, and she was never coming back.

She declared these things in order to Christopher, who let out an audible sigh on the other end. "Of course, Maggie. You can come stay on the farm. You don't have to work at all."

"No," said Maggie. "No. I mean, thanks for the offer. But actually, I've been thinking about a career change."

"What's that?"

"I'm thinking I'll get into Alaskan fishing work. I hear it's honest work, and good pay. You know anyone who wants to buy a condo?"

Christopher was briefly struck speechless at this declaration, and Maggie could just see him running his hands through his hair in confusion on the other end of the line.

"Also, my head hurts. Did you know they put staples in it?"

"Maggie, you have a concussion." Christopher laughed. "Don't sign any contracts for Alaskan fishing just yet."

"Concussion?" Maggie reached up and confirmed the presence of the staples again. "Yeah, I guess I probably do. But also I think I've never been thinking more clearly."

Maggie thought of the IUD brochure from years ago. *This is my baby, now.* She'd laughed at it back then, but perhaps those IUD marketers had seen right through her. This job had been her baby, and it had taken all of her vital forces and converted them into hair loss and anemia and self-sacrifice and sleepless nights like a real baby would. She remembered too how in med school, on her obstetrics rotation, she'd been tasked with teaching young mothers the following principle before they left the hospital:

Sometimes your baby will cry. It will cry, and cry, and cry, and cry, and cry and cry, and cry. And you will think it is your responsibility to stop the crying, to soothe the baby, to make things right. And so you feed it, and you change it, and you swaddle it, and you swing it, and bounce it, and you swing it a little harder, and you bounce it a little harder, and you swaddle it a little tighter, and you turn the white noise on a little louder, and you do all these things one after another after another, and sometimes the baby will still cry, and cry, and cry, and so you too will cry with it, as you swaddle impossibly tight and bounce impossibly hard and swing past the point of safety. And just at the moment when you think to yourself — perhaps I will just shake this baby! Just a little! Just to let him know I mean business! — you should stop and set the baby down, and back away slowly, and shut the door, and just leave. You should say — see you later, baby. You will be fine without me for a little while. Why don't you just cry yourself to sleep.

So Maggie hung up the phone, gathered her things, put on a surgical mask, and peeked out the door to find a clear path to the exit. She walked as confidently as she could, using her hospital badge to open the automated double doors, and she walked through them and then through the lobby and then through the other exit doors, and then she hung right to take the path around the backside of the hospital where a wide lookout platform stood on the waterfront side of the hospital. When she got there, she walked right to the edge, feeling that spaghetti feeling in her legs she would get at heights, the one that also came along with a weird impulse to throw herself over the ledge, an impulse she had yet to follow, and would still not follow today.

Instead, she took the hospital badge out of her bag, gripped it like one would a baseball, and she wound her arm up and threw it as high and as far as she could, watching its lanyard flutter in the wind, its two plastic rectangles spreading out like wings and catching a jet stream, circling in a way that made it look for all the world like a bird, traveling in tight spirals down, down, down, until it cleared the tree line and disappeared from view, right past the bright blue hammock slung in the trees on the hillside. *Perfect shot,* she thought.

After it was gone, she followed an impulse to head toward the tram, which was filling with tourists aiming for a sunset ride.

Through the glass above her a pink sky spread out to the horizon, and the usual tingling in her legs was replaced by warmth and gravity as the doors closed and the tram departed.

Whoooa, said a mother happily to her wide-eyed toddler as the ground beneath them seemed to disappear.

Whooooooa, said the toddler in return, raising his tiny hands above his head as if on a roller coaster. His wide eyes made contact with Maggie's and reiterated: *whooooa!*

Whooooa, Maggie reciprocated with a smile before reaching her own hands to the sky. *Whoa,* she said as her body then rocketed out of the top of the car, shattering its plexiglass ceiling and launching into the sky above, reaching an apex just as a time-traveling pterodactyl swooped down to catch her in its mouth before flying out to sea. This time, though, the pterodactyl didn't dive down to drown her. This time, the pterodactyl hung a wide right to go north, headed for Alaska.

Acknowledgments

Sincere thanks to the friends and colleagues who offered their time and encouragement as readers of the early drafts of this book. Thanks also to Desert Ink Editorial for editorial support.

Most of all, thank you to the thoughtful humanitarian leaders who designed our current healthcare system, you truly are the real MVPs. I couldn't have written this book without you.

About the Author

L.B. Cameron, MD is a real human doctor. Until such time as human doctors become relics kept only in museums dedicated to outdated technology, Dr. Cameron will be found providing outpatient primary care services to a panel of truly wonderful people who manage to make the hassles of modern medicine worthwhile.

L.B. Cameron can reluctantly be found on social media (Substack, Bluesky) as @realhumandoctormd.